IN VITRO FERTILIZATION – INNOVATIVE CLINICAL AND LABORATORY ASPECTS

Edited by **Shevach Friedler**

In Vitro Fertilization – Innovative Clinical and Laboratory Aspects
Edited by Shevach Friedler

Published by InTech

Janeza Trdine 9, 51000 Rijeka, Croatia

Publishing Process Manager Martina Blecic

Technical Editor Teodora Smiljanic

Cover Designer InTech Design Team

Additional hard copies can be obtained from orders@intechopen.com

In Vitro Fertilization – Innovative Clinical and Laboratory Aspects,
Edited by Shevach Friedler
p. cm.
ISBN 978-953-51-0503-9

For EU product safety concerns:
IN TECH d.o.o., Prolaz Marije Krucifikse Kozulić 3, 51000 Rijeka, Croatia,
info@intechopen.com or visit our website at intechopen.com.

Meet the editor

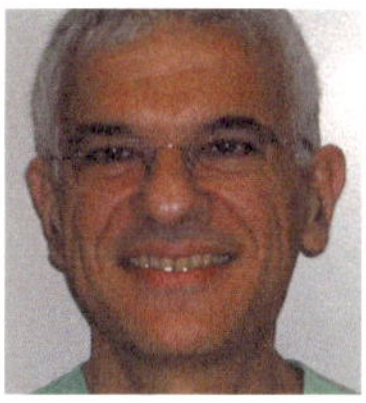

Professor Shevach Friedler is an associate professor at the Sackler School of Medicine, Tel-Aviv University and a senior physician at the Infertility and In-Vitro Fertilization Unit, at Assaf-Harofeh Medical Center, Israel, a university affiliated IVF unit, treating over 1000 IVF/ICSI cycles per year. He is also the director of the male and female infertility clinic of Kupat Cholim Meuchedet, Tel-Aviv. Prof. Friedler obtained his M.D.degree at the Medical faculty of the Hebrew University of Jerusalem. Following residency in Obstetrics and Gynecology in Jerusalem, he has done fellowship in Reproductive Endocrinology at Stanford University, California, USA. For the last twenty years he works in the field of infertility and in vitro fertilization. His scientific interests include infertility both male and female. He has authored over 85 publications including original articles, case reports, chapters in books and more, dealing with various aspects of infertility treatments, hysteroscopy, several pioneering papers concerning surgical sperm retrieval in azoospermic patients as well as different treatment modalities in in-vitro fertilization especially focusing on means improving implantation.

Contents

Preface

No doubt that one of the major advancements in the field of medicine in the last millennium, include the introduction of in-vitro fertilization and embryo transfer, to alleviate female and male infertility. Prof. Robert Edwards, the 2010 Nobel laureate in medicine represents this field. Cambridge physiologist Prof Edwards, now 85, and the late Patrick Steptoe, a gynecologic surgeon, developed IVF technology in which oocytes are fertilized outside the body and implanted in the uterine cavity. The groundbreaking work led to the birth of the world's first test tube baby, Louise Brown, in 1978. Today this technology has affected the lives of millions of infertile patients. The pioneering and inspirational work that started in the early '60s led to a breakthrough that has enhanced the lives of millions of people worldwide resulting in the birth of more than 3 million babies.

Since then, there was not a dull moment in the advancements and developments in this field. Mentioning just a few, includes embryo cryopreservation, a technology that allows preservation of surplus embryos, to be used after the fresh cycle, reducing the need of the patients to undergo another cycle of controlled ovarian hyperstimulation and oocyte retrieval, oocyte cryopreservation enabling to revolutionize the field of egg donation which enables women without fertilizable oocytes to fulfill their wish for conception and delivery. The introduction of Intracytoplasmic Sperm Injection revolutionized the treatment possibilities of male infertile patients allowing patients suffering from severe OTA and even azoospermia, to father a child. Although the field of ART exists now for more than three decades, in many of its practical aspects there is no consensus and continuing basic and clinical research relevant to the various aspects of this field contribute to its improvement.

Presently, the basic routines that IVF-ET treatments are well known to those involved in the field of reproductive medicine. In this book we present a variety of chapters expressing new and exciting data relevant to various aspects of this field, indicating the vast potential of innovations in the variable parts that comprise the puzzle of this treatment's methodology.

The first chapter relates to new aspects of the treatment protocols used for COH for IVF, specifically considering the role of low dose hCG in the late follicular phase of COH protocol. In the following chapter light is shed upon the importance of premature progesterone rise during COH, investigating the endometrial gene expression affected by it that may lead to impairment of uterine receptivity. The improvements in the instrumentation and technical ability of the new ultrasound machinery had a serious impact on the role of ultrasound in the evaluation of uterine receptivity as well as establishing the new standard of guided embryo transfer. This will be presented in our third chapter. In our fourth chapter we present a current update on the variable methods of sperm selection for IVF, including the newest ideas in this expertise. Current data indicate the importance of the preimplantation development of embryos, that may affect not only their implantation potential but also their health during their lifespan. Using in vitro fertilized bovine embryos as a mammalian model, the fifth chapter presents some histone modifications marks observed during embryonic genomic activation and how their monitoring can provide useful information about early embryo development. IVF offers hope to couples and women who might not otherwise achieve pregnancy, but there are risks which are not elucidated yet. The sixth chapter presents insights from gene expression studies during preimpantation development , essential for the evaluation of IVF safety. In our seventh chapter we present an overview on one of the newest advancement in the field of IVF. Namely, the introduction of oocyte cryopreservation by vitrification, is a methodology that may revolutionize the field of oocyte donation and fertility potential preservation. A concise overview regarding current knowledge of Preimplantation genetic testing is presented in our last chapter, presenting the current technique of PGD and PGS as well as and its future prospects using cutting edge genomic technologies allowing to prevent inherited genetic disorders.

This book is a result of collaborative work of an international group of professionals dedicated to contribute to the advancement of our knowledge that invested their time and effort in contributing their chapters. We hope that this book, presenting current new aspects pertaining to the variable aspects of the steps leading to a more effective and safer IVF, will have the ability to challenge and satisfy the curiosity of the variable potential readers seeking to enrich their knowledge in the challenging field of IVF.

Prof. Shevach Friedler
The Sackler School of Medicine, Tel Aviv University, Ramat Aviv, Israel

Part 1

Innovative Clinical Aspects of IVF

1

The Role of Low-Dose hCG[1] in the Late Follicular Phase of Controlled Ovarian Hyper Stimulation (COH) Protocols

Mahnaz Ashrafi[1,2] and Kiandokht Kiani[2]
[1]*Department of Obstetrics & Gynecology, Shahid Akbarabadi Hospital, Tehran University of Medical Sciences, Tehran,*
[2]*Department of Endocrinology and Female infertility, Reproductive Biomedicine Research Centre, Royan Institute for Reproductive Biomedicine, ACECR, Tehran, Iran*

1. Introduction

Controlled ovarian hyper-stimulation (COH) is one of the most important stages in ART treatments. The main goal of COH is to achieve efficient follicle numbers without compromising oocyte quality.

During the natural ovarian cycle, different pituitary hormones are responsible for follicle recruitment and growth. In the early follicular phase, follicle stimulating hormone (FSH) is responsible for early follicular growth and development. However, in the middle or late phase, reduction in FSH levels will occur and LH gains the more important role. The more COH protocol can mimic the natural hormonal situations, the more efficacious it will be.

In most infertile women, the administration of exogenous FSH[2] alone is usually sufficient for ovarian stimulation. In these patients, dominant follicles have LH receptors in addition to FSH ones and therefore can respond to endogenous LH. However, subgroups of cases either do not respond or over-respond to FSH. These patients may benefit from LH[3] activity supplementation during their mid or late follicular phase.

Different studies have found that LH activity supplementation may lead to improved outcome in patients over the age of 35, patients with initial abnormal response to recombinant human FSH (r-hFSH), and those at risk for poor ovarian response (Alviggi et al., 2006). In patients beyond 35 years, the addition of LH in form of human menopausal gonadotropin (hMG) to r-FSH regimen may only improve the ovarian response but does not improve overall pregnancy rates (Sohrabvand et al., 2010).

On the other hand, LH components induce the local production of various molecules such as inhibin B and IGF-1[4] from granulose cells and these factors in turn promote the growth of

---

[1] Human Chorionic Gonadotropin
[2] Follicle Stimulating Hormone
[3] Luteinizing Hormone
[4] Insulin growth factor 1

granulose cells and regulate oocyte maturation (Alviggi et al., 2006). LH is also secreted in the theca compartment and induces androgen production. Then these theca-driving androgens are converted into estradiol by aromatize enzymes (Hillier et al., 1994). These mechanisms may have an important role in the improvement of oocyte quality and LH or hCG supplementation could be a successful method for achieving the physiologic conditions for follicle growth.

Different sources of LH activity including hMG, recombinant LH and low-dose hCG are accessible. HCG is a normal natural analogue of LH. It selectively binds to LH receptors and exerts the same actions as LH (Ross 1977). It has a longer half-life than LH (Nargand et al., 2006). HCG is able to occupy LH receptors for more than 24 hours and allow stable stimulation of the LH receptors (Damewood et al., 1989). HCG is at least six times more potent than LH (Stokman et al., 1993; The European LH Study group, 2001). In other words, 200 IU hCG is equal to 1200 IU LH. It is also less expensive than recombinant FSH or hMG (Fillicori et al., 2002; Filicori et al., 2005a).

A novel gonadotropin protocol for ovarian stimulation adds low-dose hCG (50- 200 IU) in the late follicular phase (Filicori et al., 2002a; Filicori et al., 2002b; Filicori et al., 2005a; Lee et al., 2005; Sullivan et al., 1999). This component can be used alone to complete controlled ovarian stimulation (Filicori et al., 2005a). Usage of it in the late stage of ovarian stimulation (after the follicles reach≥ 12 mm) reduces gonadotropin consumption while the fertilization outcome is comparable (Filicori et al., 2005; Ashrafi et al., 2011). Furthermore this regimen reduces the number of small pre-ovulatory follicles which could reduce the risk of OHSS[5] (Fillicori et al., 2005). Adequate ovarian hormonal levels (Fillicori et al., 2005a; Branigan et al., 2005), oocyte maturation (Branigan et al., 2005), avoidance of a premature LH surge (Fillicori et al., 2005a; Branigan et al., 2005), and increased pregnancy rate (Fillicori et al., 1999; Filicori et al., 2001) are the other benefits of this regimen. This protocol also reduces the stimulation duration and the dose of exogenous FSH administration (Filicori et al., 2005a); therefore it can minimize the patient costs. HCG might also affect endometrial function, stimulate endometrial growth and maturation and enhance the endometrial angiogenesis. These effects could extend the angiogenesis. These results could lengthen the implantation window (Fillicori et al., 2005a). Tesarik et al. (2003) showed that the administration of hCG to oocyte recipients increased the endometrial thickness on the day of embryo transfer and improved the implantation rate. Adding the low-dose hCG in ovarian stimulation regimens in PCOS patients has been associated with fewer immature oocytes (Ashrafi et al., 2011).

Compounds containing LH activity have different risks and benefits. It is believed that LH has a central role in mono-follicular selection and dominance in the physiological ovulatory cycle (Fillicori et al., 2005a; Filicori et al., 2002c). Mono-folliculogenesis is ideal for intrauterine insemination (IUI), but not for IVF/ICSI treatments. In addition, LH may exert a deleterious effect on controlled ovarian stimulation. Unnecessary elevated levels of LH during the pre-ovulatory period may also negatively influence post-ovulatory events such as conception and implantation (Chappel & Howles, 1991). In addition, because hCG is at least six times more potent than LH, there is a concern that this might result in premature luteinization of the follicle.

[5] Ovarian Hyper-stimulation Syndrome

2. Indications of LH or hCG in ovarian stimulation cycles

As mentioned before, the use of low-dose hCG leads to suitable follicle growth and prevention of OHSS by small follicle atresia. Therefore, the application of LH or low-dose hCG in the late follicular phase could be divided to two parts.

2.1 LH supplementation could be used for accelerating leading follicle development

2.1.1 In patients over 35 years of age

Women, of advanced reproductive age, have low follicular recruitment. These patients also have a low number of functional LH receptors and may have low biological activity of endogenous LH (Mitchell et al., 1995; Vihko et al., 1996). In women aged over 35 undergoing intra cytoplasmic sperm injection (ICSI), LH administration led to improved outcomes (Humaidan et al., 2004; Marrs et al., 2004).

Ovarian paracrine activity also decreases with age (Hurwitz and Santoro, 2004). These paracrine variables including growth factors and cytokines may cause adequate follicular growth and steroidogenesis even when LH concentrations are very low (Alviggi et al., 2006).

2.1.2 In poor ovarian responders with GnRH antagonist protocols

In patients treated with GnRH[6] antagonists, a dramatic decline in serum concentrations of both LH and estradiol usually occurs after administration of the drug. Therefore follicles are deprived of their LH substances (Alviggi et al., 2006). A stimulation regimen consisting of GnRH-antagonist and exogenous LH in normal responders increases estradiol production but has no significant effect on improvement of IVF outcomes (Cedrin-Durnerin et al., 2004; Griesinger et al., 2005). However, this regimen is useful for women at risk for poor ovarian response (patients with less than four follicles in prior cycles and/or with basal FSH concentrations of more than 10 IU/L) (De placido et al., 2006).

2.2 LH supplementation could be used for patients with a tendency to over-respond (hyper stimulate) with standard FSH stimulation

Some patients over-respond to FSH administration and lowering of FSH can also lead to follicular growth disruption. In these patients low-dose hCG substitution could be a useful method.

2.2.1 In patients with polycystic ovarian syndrome

Women with polycystic ovarian syndrome (PCOS) are the other group that may benefit from substituting LH for FSH in the late follicular phase. They often have multi-follicular development during ovarian stimulation and are at risk for ovarian hyper-stimulation syndrome (OHSS) or multiple pregnancy. LH activity supplementation would permit the more mature follicles to continue to develop while the less mature follicles would undergo atresia due to insufficient FSH stimulation (Zelenik & Hillier, 1984; Fillicori et al., 2002). This is because the more mature follicles have acquired the adequate amount of LH receptors during the intermediate follicular phase (Fillicori et al., 2003 a,b).

---

[6] Gonadotropin releasing hormone

In our research, we assessed the effect of two low-dose hCG regimens on folliculogenesis and cycle outcome in PCOS patients and these regimens were compared with r-FSH alone. Stimulation protocol for all the patients was according to the standard long protocol (Madani et al., 2009). Gonadotropin stimulation commenced 14 days following subcutaneous GnRH agonist injection with recombinant FSH (Gonal F, Serono, Switzerland), 150 IU daily. In group B, ovarian priming with r-FSH[7] was reduced to 75 IU once the lead follicle reached 14 mm in mean diameter and low-dose hCG (100 IU/day) was administered and continued until at least two to three follicles with a mean diameter of ≥17 mm were achieved. In group C, ovarian stimulation with r-FSH was discontinued and low- dose hCG (200 IU/day) was administered when the lead follicle reached 14 mm in mean diameter and continued until at least 2–3 follicles with a mean diameter of 17 mm were achieved.

We found that the substitution of hCG for r-FSH during controlled ovarian stimulation in infertile women with PCOS reduced the rates of immature oocytes and OHSS while yielding comparable fertility outcomes, since follicles in women with PCOS, as with follicles in eumenorrheic women, become LH responsive as they mature. We also observed lower gonadotropin consumption following the addition low-dose hCG in the late follicular phase in PCOS patients (Ashrafi et al., 2011).

3. Low-dose hCG starting time

Low-dose hCG supplementation could be used in most ART protocols. However, the start time of hCG administration and discontinuation or decreasing of FSH are two important issues. In most trials, the administration of low-dose hCG was started during the middle or late follicular phase or when the follicle reached a size of more than 10 mm. In these conditions receptors for LH or hCG on the granulose cells are capable of supporting continued growth of the follicles in the absence of FSH administration (Filicori et al., 2005b). Low-dose hCG has also been started at the time of beginning stimulation with r-FSH (Van horn et al. 2007).

4. Low-dose hCG administration in assisted reproductive technologies

The addition of low-dose hCG has been used in different protocols:

4.1 In patients undergoing ovarian stimulation for timed intercourse and intra uterine insemination (IUI)

The main aim of ovarian stimulation in IUI cycles is mono follicular development. Ovarian stimulation regimens containing the FSH alone or combining the FSH and LH usually cause multi-follicular development. The low-dose hCG supplementation after the FSH priming may reduce the number of developing follicles (Fillicori et al., 2002a; 2002c; 2003a).

This regimen is also useful for patients who have previously failed to ovulate with clomiphen citrate. Branigan et al. (2006) in their RCT evaluated the effect of the low dose-hCG in previously anovulatory patients on clomiphen citrate (CC) alone. These patients underwent ovarian stimulation with CC at the 100 mg dose for timed intercourse in their

---

[7] Recombinant FSH

previous cycles and failed to ovulate on this regimen. They found that the use of low dose-hCG (200IU) after CC in the late follicular phase resulted in good ovulation and pregnancy rates in these patients.

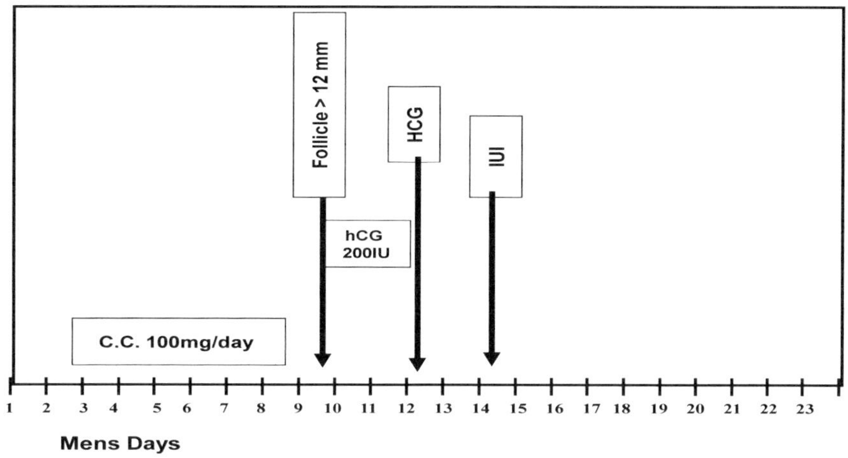

Fig. 1. Clomiphen Citrate + Low-dose hCG

4.2 Low dose hCG administration in conjunction with GnRH antagonists

The use of GnRH antagonist instead of GnRH agonist in IVF cycles has increased in recent years. Different strategies could be used for GnRh antagonist administration. A single depot maybe used on cycle stimulation day eight or nine which lasts four days and is sufficient to prevent the LH surge in 80%of women (Olivennes et al., 1998). Alternatively, multiple small doses may be used daily from cycle day six as a fixed order, or when the leading follicle has reached a 14 mm diameter in a more flexible manner, until the hCG trigger.

This protocol has some benefits. For example, it can lead to immediate pituitary suppression (Tarlatzis et al., 2006). The decreasing of OHSS, lowering the gonadotropin consumption, and avoidance of the gonadotropin flare are the other benefits of this protocol (Tarlatzis et al., 2006; Griesinger et al., 2010). However, the LH level in the GnRH antagonist protocol decreases (Duijkers et al., 1998; Griesinger et al., 2010) and this may negatively affect implantation or pregnancy rate (Esposito et al., 2001). LH secretion is necessary for appropriate follicular and endometrial development (Shoham et al., 2008; Kaufmann et al., 2007).

Adding the low-dose hCG to the GnRH antagonist protocol may compensate for its shortcomings. It can be added to all types of GnRH antagonist protocols which have been mentioned before. It may improve the implantation and live birth rates in patients with low LH levels (Propst et al., 2011). Low-dose hCG supplementation results in higher estradiol secretion of granulose cells and cumulous cell expansion that causes better oocyte maturation rates and endometrial preparation (Cedrin-Durnerin et al., 2004; Ben-Ami et al., 2009). The effect of hCG on endometrium regulation and implantation has been suggested in previous studies (Filicori et al., 2005; Cameo et al., 2006; d'Hauterive et al., 2007). LH administration can increase the LH/hCG receptors during the pre-implantation window and also prevents apoptosis of the endometrial stromal cells (Lovely et al., 2005; Jasinska et al., 2006).

Serafini et al. (2006) showed that using a low-dose hCG protocol along with a GnRH antagonist treatment in normal ovarian responders avoids premature ovulation, and OHSS. It also decreases the total dose of recombinant FSH. This protocol permitted follicles and oocytes to develop fully and aided normal fertilization along with the generation of top-quality embryos and establishment of clinical pregnancies.

Van Horne et al., (2007) also found a reduction in r-FSH requirements and an average cost saving of $600 per cycle in patients who used low-dose hCG supplementation in the GnRH antagonist cycles. These patients had similar implantation and pregnancy rates compared with GnRH antagonist cycles that used r-FSH alone.

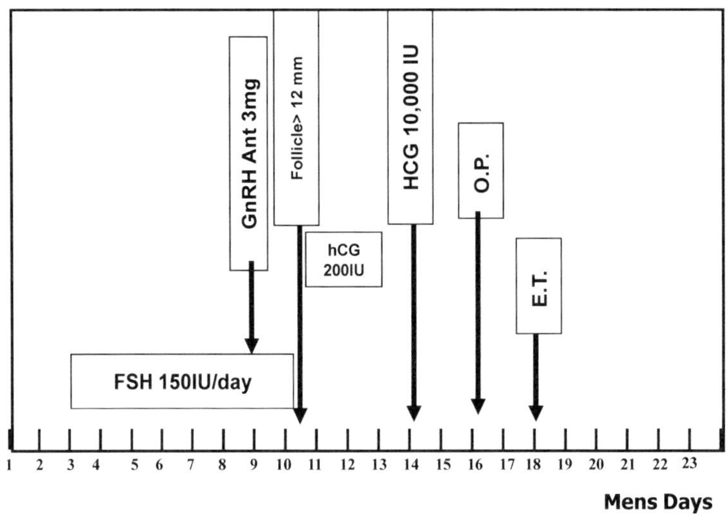

Fig. 2. GnRH antagonist (Single Dose) + Low dose hCG

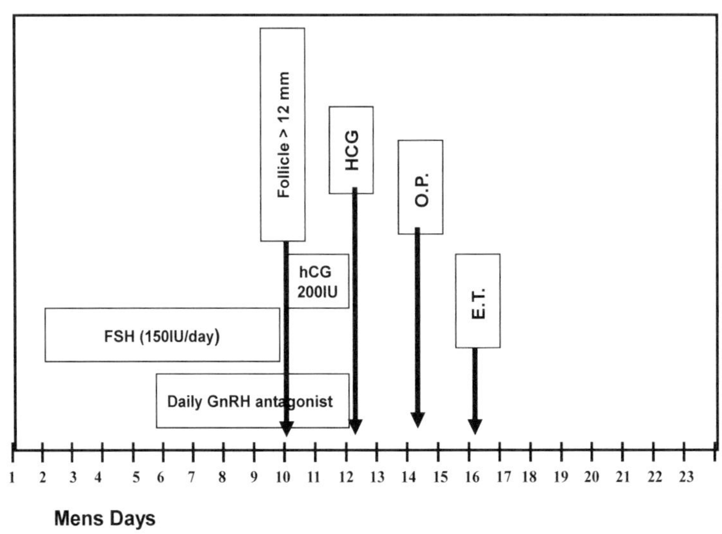

Fig. 3. GnRH antagonist (Multiple Dose) + Low dose hCG

4.3 Low-dose hCG administration in women undergoing IVF cycles down-regulated with GnRH agonists

There are two protocols for the usage of GnRH agonists in ART cycles.

1. Long protocol

For this protocol, all patients usually receive Buserelin 500 μgr (0.5 mg) via subcutaneous injection starting on day 21 of their menstrual cycles. Down-regulation is confirmed by a linear endometrium in ultrasonography (endometrium below 3 mm) and suppressed ovaries by serum estradiol concentration< 60 pg/ml. Gonadotropin stimulation commence 14 days following subcutaneous GnRH agonist injection with recombinant FSH, 150 IU daily. The dose of GnRH agonist will be decreased at this moment (to 200 μgr). The dose and duration of FSH treatment are adjusted by monitoring follicular development with ultrasound and estradiol levels. FSH administration is discontinued and low-dose hCG is added when the lead follicle reached to more than 12 mm. The goal of ovarian stimulation is to achieve at least two ovarian follicles with a mean diameter of ≥17 mm on the day of hCG administration. Then, 10,000 IU of hCG is administered and oocyte retrieval is performed 34-36 hours later.

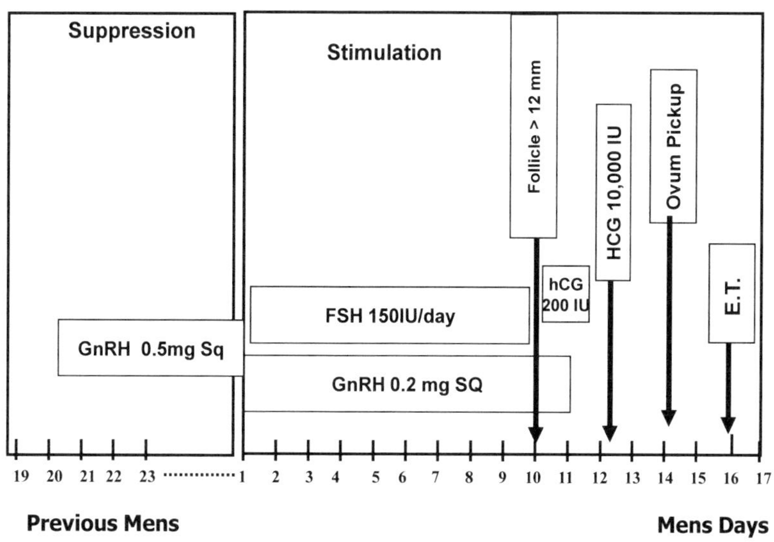

Fig. 4. GnRH Agonist Long Protocol+ 200 IU Low Dose hCG

2. Short protocol

The short or flare protocol employs the agonist-induced flare-up of endogenous FSH to stimulate the ovary in addition to exogenous FSH administration. The agonist is started on day two of the cycle with gonadotrophins on day three. Follicular growth takes 10-12 days which is adequate to down-regulate the pituitary gland and prevent a premature LH surge (Daya, 2000). The administration of recombinant FSH, 150 IU daily will be discontinued when the lead follicle reached to more than 12 mm. In this condition low dose hCG is added. The goal of ovarian stimulation is to achieve an average of two ovarian follicles with a mean diameter of ≥17 mm on the day of hCG administration. Then, 10,000 IU of hCG is administered and oocyte retrieval is performed 34–36 h later.

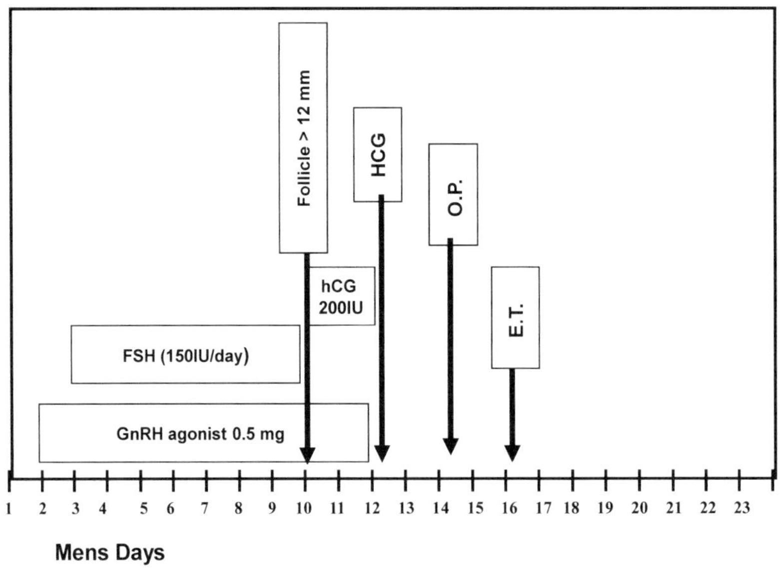

Fig. 5. GnRH Agonist Short Protocol+ 200 IU Low Dose hCG

5. Conclusion

Use of low-dose hCG in the mid to late follicular phase of COH provides these results:

1. This protocol provides adequate ovarian estradiol secretion, oocyte maturation, and acceptable fertilization rates.
2. This protocol provides significant reduction of FSH dosage and reduced cost of treatment.
3. This protocol has no adverse effects on the number of oocyte retrieved and pregnancy rate but can prevent the occurrence of OHSS with a reduced number of follicles and cancelled cycles.

6. References

Alviggi C., Clarizia R., Mollo A., Ranieri A., & De Placido G. (2006). Outlook: who needs LH in ovarian stimulation? *Reproductive Biomedicine Online,* Vol.12, No.5, pp. 599-607.

Ashrafi M., Kiani K., Ghasemi A., Rastegar F., & Nabavi M. (2011). The effect of low dose human chorionic gonadotropin on follicular response and oocyte maturation in PCOS patients undergoing IVF cycles: a randomized clinical trial of efficacy and safety. *Archives of Gynecology and Obstetrics,* Vol. 284, No.6, pp.1431-1438.

Ben-Ami I., Armon L., Freimann S., Strassburger D., Ron-El R., & Amsterdam A.(2009). EGF-like growth factors as LH mediators in the human corpus luteum. *Human Reproduction,* Vol. 24, No. 1, pp.176–184.

Branigan EF., & Estes A. (2005). Use of micro-dose human chorionic gonadotropin (hCG) after clomiphene citrate (CC) to complete folliculogenesis in previous CC-resistant anovulation. *American Journal of Obstetrics and Gynecology*, Vol. 192, No.6, pp. 1890-1894.

Cédrin-Durnerin I., Grange-Dujardin D., Laffy A., Parneix I., Massin N., Galey J., Théron L., Wolf JP., Conord C., Clément P., Jayot S., & Hugues JN. (2004). Recombinant human LH supplementation during GnRH antagonist administration in IVF/ICSI cycles: a prospective randomized study. *Human Reproduction*. Vol. 19, No. 9, pp. 1979-1984.

Chappel SC. &Howles C. (1991). Reevaluation of the roles of luteinizing hormones and follicle-stimulating hormone in the ovulatory process. *Human Reproduction*. Vol. 6, No.9, pp. 1206–1212.

Damewood MD., Shen W., Zacur HA., Schlaff WD., Rock JA., & Wallach EE. (1989). Disappearance of exogenously administered human chorionic gonadotropin. *Fertility and Sterility*. Vol. 52, No.3, pp. 398-400.

Daya S. (2000). Gonadotropin releasing hormone agonist protocols for pituitary desensitization in in vitro fertilization and gamete intrafallopian transfer cycles. *Cochrane Database of Systematic Reviews*. Vol. 2, CD001299.

De Placido G., Mollo A., Clarizia R., Strina I., Conforti S., & Alviggi C. (2006). Gonadotropin-releasing hormone (GnRH) antagonist plus recombinant luteinizing hormone vs. a standard GnRH agonist short protocol in patients at risk for poor ovarian response. Fertility and Sterility. Vol. 85, No. 1, pp. 247-250.

Duijkers IJM., Klipping C., Willemsen WNP., Krone D., Schneider E., Niebch G., & Hermann R. Single and multiple dose pharmacokinetics and pharmacodynamics of the gonadotrophin-releasing hormone antagonist Cetrorelix in healthy female volunteers. (1989). *Human Reproduction*. Vol. 13, No. 9, pp.2392–2398.

Filicori M., Cognigni GE., & Ciampaglia W. (2003b). What clinical evidence for an LH ceiling? *Human Reproduction*. Vol. 18, No. 7, pp: 1556-1557.

Filicori M., Cognigni GE., Gamberini E., Parmegiani L., Troilo E., & Roset B. (2005a). Efficacy of low-dose human chorionic gonadotropin alone to complete controlled ovarian stimulation. *Fertility and Sterility*. Vol. 84, No. 2, pp. 394-401.

Filicori M., Cognigni GE., Pocognoli P., Ciampaglia W., & Bernardi S.(2003a). Current concepts and novel applications of LH activity in ovarian stimulation. *Trends in Endocrinology and Metabolism*. Vol. 14, No. 6, pp. 267-273.

Filicori M., Cognigni GE., Samara A., Melappioni S., Perri T., Cantelli B., Parmegiani L., Pelusi G., DeAloysio D. (2002c). The use of LH activity to drive folliculogenesis: exploring uncharted territories in ovulation induction. *Human Reproduction Update*. Vol. 8, No. 6, pp. 543–557.

Filicori M., Cognigni GE., Tabarelli C., Pocognoli P., Taraborrelli S., Spettoli D., & Ciampaglia W. (2002a). Stimulation and growth of antral ovarian follicles by selective LH activity administration in women. *The Journal of Clinical Endocrinology and Metabolism*. Vol. 87, No. 3, pp. 1156-1161.

Filicori M., Cognigni GE., Taraborrelli S., Parmegiani L., Bernardi S., & Ciampaglia W. (2002b). Intracytoplasmic sperm injection pregnancy after low-dose human chorionic gonadotropin alone to support ovarian folliculogenesis. *Fertility and Sterility*. Vol. 78, No. 2, pp. 414-416.

Filicori M., Cognigni GE., Taraborrelli S., Spettoli D., Ciampaglia W., de Fatis CT., Pocognoli P. (1999). Luteinizing hormone activity supplementation enhances follicle-stimulating hormone efficacy and improves ovulation induction outcome. *The Journal of Clinical Endocrinology and Metabolism*. Vol. 84, No. 8, pp. 2659 -2663.

Filicori M., Cognigni GE., Taraborrelli S., Spettoli D., Ciampaglia W., Tabarelli de Fatis C., Pocognoli P., Cantelli B., & Boschi S. (2001). Luteinizing hormone activity in menotropins optimizes folliculogenesis and treatment in controlled ovarian stimulation. *The Journal of Clinical Endocrinology and Metabolism*. Vol. 86, No. 1, pp.337- 343.

Filicori M., Fazleabas AT., Huhtaniemi I., Licht P., Rao ChV., Tesarik J., & Zygmunt M.(2005b). Novel concepts of human chorionic gonadotropin: reproductive system interactions and potential in the management of infertility. *Fertility and Sterility*. Vol. 84, No. 2, pp. 275-284.

Griesinger G. Ovarian hyperstimulation syndrome prevention strategies: use of gonadotropin-releasing hormone antagonists. (2010). Seminars in Reproductive Medicine. Vol.28, No. 6, pp. 493–499.

Griesinger G., Schultze-Mosgau A., Dafopoulos K., Schroeder A., Schroer A., von Otte S., Hornung D., Diedrich K., & Felberbaum R. (2005). Recombinant luteinizing hormone supplementation to recombinant follicle-stimulating hormone induced ovarian hyperstimulation in the GnRH-antagonist multiple-dose protocol. *Human Reproduction*. Vol. 20, No. 5, pp.1200-1206.

Hillier SG., Whitelaw PF., & Smyth CD. (1994). Follicular oestrogen synthesis: the 'two-cell, two-gonadotrophin' model revisited. *Molecular and Cellular Endocrinology*. Vol. 100, No. (1-2), pp. 51-54.

Humaidan P., Bungum M., Bungum L., Yding Andersen C. (2004). Effects of recombinant LH supplementation in women undergoing assisted reproduction with GnRH agonist down-regulation and stimulation with recombinant FSH: an opening study. *Reproductive and Biomedicine Online*. Vol. 8, No. 6, pp. 635-643.

Hurwitz JM., & Santoro N. (2004). Inhibins, activins, and follistatin in the aging female and male. *Seminars in Reproductive Medicine*. Vol. 22, No. 3, pp.209-217.

Jasinska A., Strakova Z., Szmidt M., Fazleabas AT. (2006). Human chorionic gonadotropin and decidualization in vitro inhibits cytochalasin-D-induced apoptosis in cultured endometrial stromal fibroblasts. *Endocrinology*. Vol. 147, No. 9, pp. 4112–4121.

Kaufmann R., Dunn R., Vaughn T., Hughes G., O'Brien F., Hemsey G., Thomson B., & O'Dea LS. (2007). Recombinant human luteinizing hormone, lutropin alfa, for the induction of follicular development and pregnancy in profoundly gonadotrophin-deficient women. *Clinical Endocrinology*. Vol. 67, No. 4, pp.563–569.

Lee KL., Couchman GM., & Walmer DK. (2005). Successful pregnancies in patients with estrogenic anovulation after low-dose human chorionic gonadotropin therapy alone following hMG for controlled ovarian hyperstimulation. *Journal of Assisted Reproduction and Genetics*. Vol. 22, No. 1, pp. 37-40.

Lovely LP., Fazleabas AT., Fritz MA., McAdams DG., Lessey BA. (2005). Prevention of endometrial apoptosis: Randomized prospective comparison of human chorionic gonadotropin versus progesterone treatment in the luteal phase. *The Journal of Clinical Endocrinology and Metabolism*. Vol. 90, No.4, pp.2351–2356.

Madani T., Ashrafi M., Abadi AB., & Kiani K. (2009). Appropriate timing of uterine cavity length measurement positively affects assisted reproduction cycle outcome. *Reproductive Biomedicine Online*. Vol. 19, No. 5, pp.734–736

Marrs R., Meldrum D., Muasher S., Schoolcraft W., Werlin L., & Kelly E. (2004). Randomized trial to compare the effect of recombinant human FSH (follitropin alfa) with or without recombinant human LH in women undergoing assisted reproduction treatment. *Reproductive Biomedicine Online*. Vol. 8, No. 2, pp. 175-182.

Mitchell R., Hollis S., Rothwell C., & Robertson WR. (1995). Age related changes in the pituitary-testicular axis in normal men; lower serum testosterone results from decreased bioactive LH drive. *Clinical Endocrinology (Oxf)*. Vol. 42, No. 5, pp. 501-507.

Olivennes F., Alvarez S., Bouchard P., Fanchin R., Salat-Baroux J. & Frydman R. (1998). The use of a GnRH antagonist (Cetrorelix) in a single dose protocol in IVF-embryo transfer: a dose finding study of 3 versus 2 mg. *Human Reproduction*. Vol. 13, No. 9, pp. 2411–2414.

Propst AM., Hill MJ., Bates GW., Palumbo M., Van Horne AK., & Retzloff MG. (2011). Low-dose human chorionic gonadotropin may improve in vitro fertilization cycle outcomes in patients with low luteinizing hormone levels after gonadotropin-releasing hormone antagonist administration. *Fertility and Sterility*. Vol. 96, No. 4, pp. 898-904.

Ross GT. Clinical relevance of research on the structure of human chorionic gonadotropin. (1977). *American Journal of Obstetrics and Gynecology*. Vol. 129, No. 7, pp. 795-808.

Serafini P., Yadid I., Motta EL., Alegretti JR., Fioravanti J., & Coslovsky M. (2006). Ovarian stimulation with daily late follicular phase administration of low-dose human chorionic gonadotropin for in vitro fertilization: a prospective, randomized trial. Fertility and Sterility. Vol. 86, No.4, pp.830–838

Shoham Z., Smith H., Yeko T., O'Brien F., Hemsey G., & O'Dea L. (2008). Recombinant LH (lutropin alfa) for the treatment of hypogonadotrophic women with profound LH deficiency: a randomized, double-blind, placebo-controlled, proof-of-efficacy study. *Clinical Endocrinology*. Vol. 69, No. 3, pp. 471–478.

Sohrabvand F., Golestan B., Kashani H., Saberi M., Haghollahi F., Maasomi M., Bagheri M. Comparison of ART outcomes between two COH protocols: Gonal-F versus Gonal-F plus HMG. *International Journal of Fertility and Sterility*. Vol. 3, No. 4, pp. 161- 164.

Stokman PG., de Leeuw R., van den Wijngaard HA., Kloosterboer HJ., Vemer HM., Sanders AL. (1993). Human chorionic gonadotropin in commercial human menopausal gonadotropin preparations. *Fertility and Sterility*. Vol. 60, No. 1, pp. 175– 178.

Sullivan MW., Stewart-Akers A., Krasnow JS., Berga SL., & Zeleznik AJ. (1999). Ovarian responses in women to recombinant follicle-stimulating hormone and luteinizing hormone (LH): a role for LH in the final stages of follicular maturation. *The Journal of Clinical Endocrinology and Metabolism*. Vol. 84, No.1, pp. 228-232.

Tarlatzis BC., Fauser BC., Kolibianakis EM., Diedrich K., & Devroey P. (2006). GnRH antagonists in ovarian stimulation for IVF. *Human Reproduction Update*. Vol. 12, No. 4, pp. 333–340.

Tesarik J., Hazout A., & Mendoza C. (2003). Luteinizing hormone affects uterine receptivity independently of ovarian function. *Reproductive Biomedicine Online*. Vol.7, No. 1, pp. 59-64.

The European Recombinant LH Study Group. (2001). Human recombinant luteinizing hormone is as effective as, but safer than, urinary human chorionic gonadotropin in inducing final follicular maturation and ovulation in in vitro fertilization procedures: results of a multicenter double-blind study. *The Journal of Clinical Endocrinology and Metabolism*. Vol. 86, No. 6, pp.2607–2618.

Van Horne AK., Bates GW Jr., Robinson RD., Arthur NJ., & Propst AM. (2007). Recombinant follicle-stimulating hormone (rFSH) supplemented with low-dose human chorionic gonadotropin compared with rFSH alone for ovarian stimulation for in vitro fertilization. *Fertility and Sterility*. Vol. 88, No. 4, pp. 1010-1013.

Vihko KK., Kujansuu E., Mörsky P., Huhtaniemi I., & Punnonen R. (1996). Gonadotropins and gonadotropin receptors during the perimenopause. *European Journal of Endocrinology*. Vol. 134, No. 3, pp. 357-361.

Zeleznik AJ., & Hillier SG. (1984). The role of gonadotropins in the selection of the preovulatory follicle. *Clinical Obstetrics and Gynecology*. Vol. 27, No. 4, pp. 927-940.

2

Gene Expression and Premature Progesterone Rise

Inge Van Vaerenbergh[1] and Christophe Blockeel[2]
[1]*Department of Pathology, UZ Brussel and Reproductive Immunology and Implantation (REIM), Vrije Universiteit Brussel, Jette,*
[2]*Centre for Reproductive Medicine, UZ Brussel / Vrije Universiteit Brussel, Jette, Belgium*

1. Introduction

In present stimulation protocols for IVF, some patients experience a rise in serum progesterone (P) concentration in the late follicular phase. Premature P rise affects about 5 to as high as 38% of IVF patients (Edelstein et al., 1990; Silverberg et al., 1991; Ubaldi et al., 1996; Bosch et al., 2003) and is associated with lower implantation and pregnancy rates. It is defined as a rise in P concentration towards the end of the follicular phase above a certain threshold, which is set arbitrarily. There is an ongoing debate about the definition of premature luteinisation, or better defined as 'premature progesterone rise', as to which threshold for premature P rise should be established (Van Vaerenbergh et al., 2011; Labarta et al., 2011). Therefore, the changes in gene expression were studied in patients with premature progesterone rise.

2. Research methods

2.1 Patients

This study was approved by the Ethics Committee of the University Hospital of the Vrije Universiteit Brussel. All patients signed an informed consent. The patients included in the study were women below 37 years of age who underwent a first or second treatment cycle of in-vitro fertilisation (IVF) with intracytoplasmic sperm injection (ICSI). Patients were excluded from the study if they requested preimplantation genetic diagnosis, had an azoospermic partner or had a serum follicle-stimulating hormone (FSH) level on day 3 of the menstrual cycle of more than 12 IU/L. A single embryo transfer policy was applied in all cycles. Patients with endometriosis ≥ stage III (AFS (American Fertility Society) classification), with PCOS (polycystic ovary syndrome; defined according to the Rotterdam 2003 criteria, Rotterdam ESHRE/ASRM-Sponsored PCOS Consensus Workshop Group, 2004) or with any other endometrial pathology were excluded from the study.

2.2 Stimulation protocol

Ovarian stimulation was performed with a median starting dose of 200 IU rec-FSH (follicle stimulating hormone, Puregon®, MSD, Oss, The Netherlands), from day 2 until day 6 of the cycle. From day 7 onwards, the dose was adjusted individually. To inhibit premature LH surge, daily GnRH-antagonist (Orgalutran® 0,25mg, MSD) was used from the morning of day 6 of stimulation. Final oocyte maturation was achieved by administration of 10 000 IU of hCG (human chorionic gonadotrophin, Pregnyl®, MSD) as soon as 3 (or more) follicles ≥ 17 mm were present. Oocyte retrieval was carried out 36 hours after hCG administration. The luteal phase was supported with 600 mg micronized progesterone (Utrogestan®, Piette, Brussels, Belgium) (Figure 1). IVF and ICSI procedures have been described in detail elsewhere (Van Landuyt et al., 2005).

Freshly ejaculated sperm was used. One or two embryos were transferred in the same cycle on day 3 or day 5 of embryo culture, according to the Belgian reimbursement law. Embryo quality was comparable between patients.

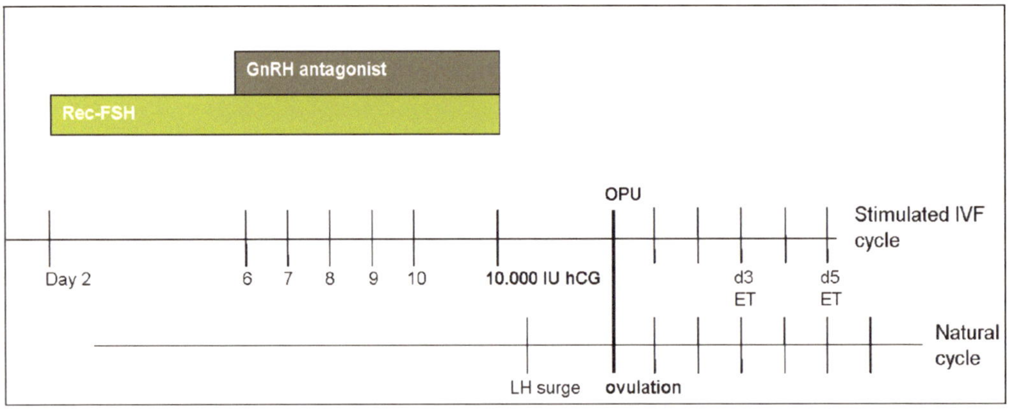

ET: embryo transfer, OPU: oocyte pick-up or oocyte retrieval.

Fig. 1. Stimulation protocol in a GnRH antagonist/rec-FSH IVF cycle. The day of oocyte retrieval in a stimulated cycle is analogous to the day of ovulation in a natural cycle.

2.3 Human uterine tissue collection

Endometrial biopsies were taken with a pipelle (Pipelle de Cornier®, Prodimed, Neuilly-en-Thelle, France) under sterile conditions on the day of oocyte retrieval. The biopsies were divided into two parts. One part of the endometrial tissue was used for classical histological analysis with haematoxylin and eosin staining. Endometrial dating was performed on all samples according to the criteria of Noyes (Noyes et al., 1950) by a pathologist, blinded for clinical outcome. The other part was snap-frozen in liquid nitrogen under sterile conditions for further RNA isolation and gene expression analysis with microarray technology, followed by validation with a more quantitative PCR.

2.4 Gene expression profiling

RNA extraction was performed using the RNeasy Mini kit (Qiagen, Valencia, CA, USA). Total RNA concentration was measured with the NanoDrop ND-1000 spectrophotometer (NanoDrop Technologies, Wilmington, DE, USA) and integrity of the RNA samples was controlled using the Agilent 2100 Bioanalyzer with the RNA 6000 Nano Kit (Agilent Technologies Inc., Palo Alto, CA, USA).

The human genome encodes for approximately 25 000 genes, however only a subset is active or expressed in any cell and the levels and timing of RNA expression regulate cellular development, differentiation and function. Microarrays are a tool to make a snapshot of the gene expression situation in a cell or tissue at a particular moment.

For the gene expression analysis, 2 µg of the total amount of isolated RNA was reverse transcribed with the SuperScript Choice System (Invitrogen, Carlsbad, CA, USA) with oligo-dT primers containing a T7 RNA polymerase promotor site (Figure 2). Then, cDNA was *in vitro* transcribed and labelled with biotin using the IVT labelling kit (Affymetrix, Santa Clara, CA, USA) followed by the fragmentation of the biotinylated cRNA. The fragmented cRNA was hybridized overnight to the Affymetrix Human Genome (HG) U133 Plus 2.0 Array (Affymetrix). This array contains more than 54 000 probe sets. Each probe set is designed to detect one specific gene or transcript. The microarray contains a redundant number of probe sets. A gene can be represented by 2 or even more than 10 probe sets. This means that about 54 000 probe sets on the Affymetrix HG U133 Plus 2.0 Array cover the whole human genome of about 20 000-30 000 genes.

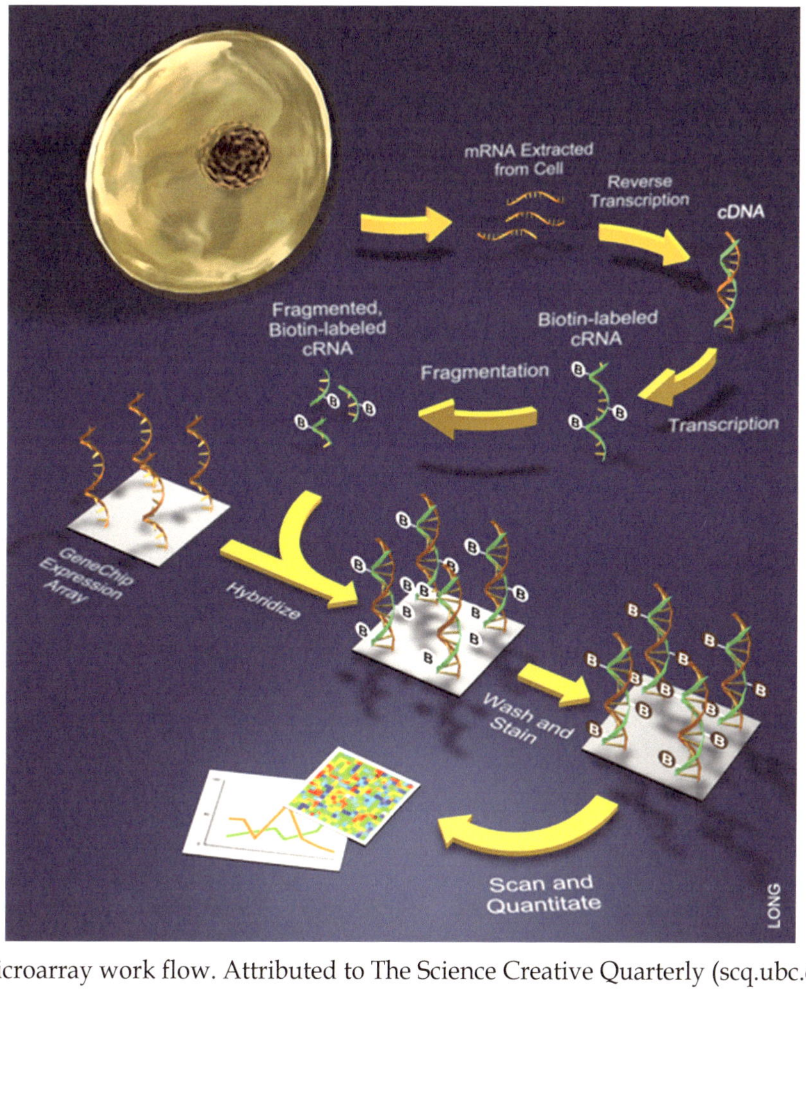

Fig. 2. Microarray work flow. Attributed to The Science Creative Quarterly (scq.ubc.ca).

2.5 Data analysis

2.5.1 Significant differential expression

Affymetrix GeneChip Operating Software (GCOS) version 1.4 with the MAS 5.0 algorithm was used to analyse the resulting image files. Transcripts were considered as differentially expressed when the following criteria were met: (i) present (P) 'calls' in all samples of the selected group; (ii) consistent (minimum in 2/3 of the comparisons) decreased or increased change in expression for pair-wise comparisons between the two selected groups; (iii) a mean absolute value of the signal log ratio (SLR) ≥ 0.5; this equals a fold change ratio (FC) of 1.4 or higher and (iv) a two-tailed unpaired Student's t-test with a significant result ($P \leq 0.05$). The data files have been deposited in NCBI's public database Gene Expression Omnibus (GEO) according to MIAME (Minimum Information About a Microarray Experiment) guidelines.

2.5.2 PCA and clustering

Principal component analysis (PCA) and hierarchical clustering was performed in an unsupervised way with GeneSpring GX software (Agilent Technologies). Principal component analysis is mainly used to visually assess the quality of replicate samples. Each point in the 3D plot represents a sample. With multiple replicates in each group, the replicates should be grouped together. If any of the biological replicates mix with another group, this sample may be further examined. PCA is a tool to visualize multidimensional data, like microarray data, into two or three dimensions. Each dimension represents a principal component (PC) with a certain percentage of variance. The percentage of variation is captured along three axes with the first axis (PCA 1) having the largest percentage of variation.

Hierarchical cluster analysis is a statistical method to group samples unsupervised in different clusters or branches of the hierarchical or condition tree. In this way, the relationships between the different groups are shown (Eisen et al., 1998). The condition tree can be displayed as a so-called 'heat map', based on the measured expression levels of the probe sets.

2.5.3 Network and pathway analysis

Further gene ontology study was performed with Ingenuity Pathways Analysis (IPA) software (Ingenuity® Systems, www.ingenuity.com, Redwood City, CA, USA) for further network and pathway analysis. A data file was uploaded that contained the gene identifiers for the differentially expressed probe sets and the corresponding expression values. Each gene identifier was mapped to its corresponding gene (object) in the Ingenuity Pathways Knowledge Base (IPKB). A log ratio threshold of 0.5 was set to identify focus genes whose expression was significantly differentially regulated. Networks of these genes were then algorithmically generated based on their connectivity in the IPKB. The networks were assigned a score, according to their relevance to the list of focus genes. Each network was arbitrarily set to have a maximum of 35 focus genes. Networks are shown as nodes and lines: nodes represent genes and lines represent the relationships between the genes (see Figure 4 in the Results section). All lines are supported by at least one reference from the literature. The intensity of the node colour indicates the degree of up- (red) or down- (green) regulation. Nodes are displayed using various shapes representing the functional class of the gene product (see legend Figure 4).

The functional analysis identified the biological functions and/or diseases that were most significant to the data set (see Figure 5). Genes from the data set that met the P-value threshold of 0.05 (Fisher's exact test) and were associated with biological functions and/or diseases in the IPKB were considered for the analysis.

Canonical pathway analysis (see Figure 6) identified the pathways most significant to the data set, based on two parameters: (i) a ratio of the number of genes from the data set that map to the pathway divided by the total number of genes that map to the canonical pathway; (ii) Fisher's exact test was used to calculate a P-value determining the probability that the association between the genes in the dataset and the canonical pathway is explained by chance alone (www.ingenuity.com/company/pdf/Citation_Guidelines_2005-09-13.pdf).

2.6 QPCR validation

Quantitative validation was performed with QPCR for selected genes. Genes were selected for validation by quantitative real-time PCR (QPCR) because of their highly significant p-value or fold change ratio (FC) and/or because more than one probe set for the same gene was significantly differentially expressed. The selection also occurred on the available literature.

A two-step real-time PCR was performed. A reverse-transcription reaction from total RNA was achieved with the High-Capacity cDNA Archive kit (Applied Biosystems, Foster City, CA, USA) following the manufacturer's protocol. The quantitative real-time PCR was performed with the TaqMan Gene Expression Assay (Applied Biosystems), containing two unlabeled primers and one TaqMan FAM dye-labelled MGB ('minor groove binding') probe. Glyceraldehyde-3-phosphate dehydrogenase (GAPDH) was chosen as the control housekeeping gene using the TaqMan Endogenous Control Assay (Applied Biosystems) containing two unlabeled primers and one TaqMan FAM dye-labelled MGB probe. Both assays are cDNA specific, since the probes span an exon junction.

All real-time PCR assays were run using the TaqMan Universal PCR Master Mix plus AmpErase UNG (Applied Biosystems) on the 7900 HT Fast System (Applied Biosystems). Thermal cycling parameters were set as follows: 2 min. at 50°C (AmpErase UNG activation), 10 min. at 95°C (AmpliTaq Gold activation), followed by 40 cycles of denaturation, annealing and extension (15 sec. at 95°C and 1 min. at 60°C, respectively). No-template and no-RT (reverse transcriptase) controls were included to verify the quality and cDNA specificity of the primers. All samples were analysed in triplicate. The relative quantification was performed by the standard curve method. For each sample, the amount of target gene and endogenous control (GAPDH) was determined from their respective standard curves. First, the target gene amount was divided by the endogenous control amount to obtain a normalized value. In a second step, the samples were normalized again to the sample with the lowest normalized expression, the calibrator sample or 1x sample. Therefore, each of the normalized values was divided by the calibrator normalized value to generate the relative expression levels. Significance was achieved when $p < 0.05$ (with t-test).

3. Results

3.1 Patient groups

The endometrial gene expression profile on the day of oocyte retrieval in rec-FSH stimulated GnRH-antagonist cycles for IVF with embryo transfer in the same cycle was studied and correlated with the serum P concentration on the day of hCG administration (Van Vaerenbergh et al., 2011). Three groups of patients (n= 14 in total) with different serum P concentrations on the day of hCG were analysed: a group with P below 0.9 ng/ml, an intermediate group with P from 1 to 1.5 ng/ml and a high concentration group with P above 1.5 ng/ml. These cut-offs were based on the recent literature (Papanikolaou et al., 2009; Venetis et al., 2007). In these articles, 0.9 ng/ml was found as the lowest threshold for P concentration and 1.5 ng/ml was found as the highest threshold. Although different cut-offs have been used over the years ranging from 0.8 to even 2 ng/ml (Hofmann et al., 1993; Ubaldi et al., 1996; Silverberg et al., 1994; Edelstein et al., 1990; Givens et al., 1994), in recent publications the upper cut-off level is set at 1.5 ng/ml.

In these three groups of patients, the patients with a clinical pregnancy (defined according to ICMART/WHO terminology, as a pregnancy diagnosed by ultrasonographic visualization of one or more gestational sacs or definitive clinical signs of pregnancy; Zegers-Hochschild et al., 2009) were observed in the low and intermediate group. No clinical pregnancies occurred when the P concentration on the day of hCG administration was above 1.5 ng/ml.

Histological dating demonstrated an advanced secretory endometrial maturation for the majority of patients (13 out of 14 or 92.8%), ranging from +day 2 (two days advanced as compared to the chronological cycle day, which is the day of oocyte retrieval, considered as day 0) to +day 4.

3.2 Gene expression

In the comparison between 3 groups, a small difference in gene expression between the first two groups was found. However, the gene expression profile from patients with high P concentration (> 1.5 ng/ml) was significantly different from the patients in the other two groups. These results were also confirmed with principal component analysis and hierarchical clustering, where a separate cluster for patients with high P concentration (> 1.5 ng/ml) was found (Figure 3a and 3b). In this way, the threshold of 1.5 ng/ml, as suggested in recent literature (Papanikolaou et al., 2009; Bosch et al., 2010), was confirmed at the molecular level.

3.3 Validation with QPCR

The results obtained with the microarray gene expression analysis have been validated for selected genes with a more quantitative real-time PCR technique. Some of the genes that were selected for validation had already known roles in the reproductive system. For example DKK3 (Dickkopf homolog 3) is a known molecule in the Wnt/ β catenin signalling pathway. Other genes that were selected for validation with QPCR were: PAPPA (pregnancy associated plasma protein A or pappalysin), PRSS23 (protease serine 23), IL17RB (interleukin 17 receptor B), and THSD4 (thrombospondin type 1 domain containing 4).

These genes all showed a significant fold change (compared between the intermediate P concentration group and the high concentration group) comparable with their fold changes obtained in the microarray experiment.

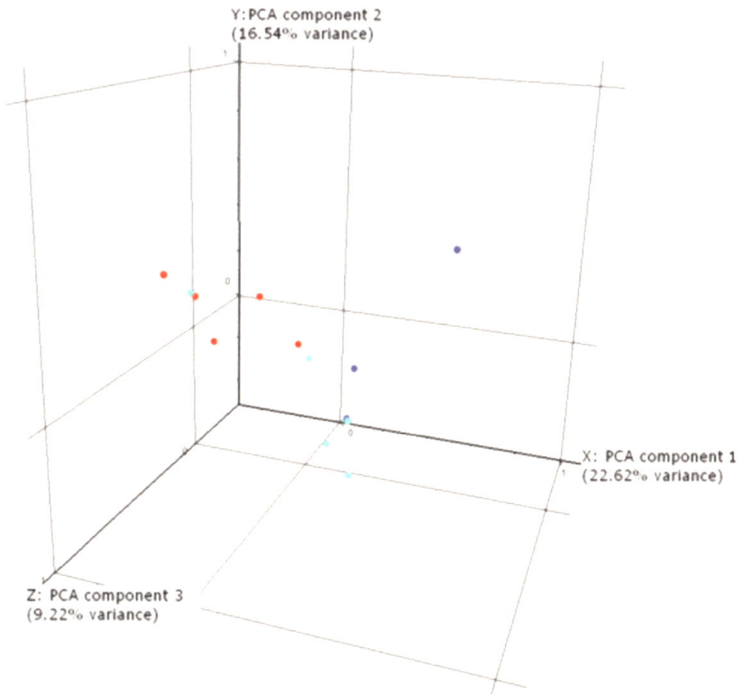

Fig. 3a. Principal component analysis (PCA) of 14 endometrial biopsies of patients with premature P rise on the day of hCG administration: low P concentration group (dark blue), an intermediate P concentration group (light blue) and high P concentration group (red).

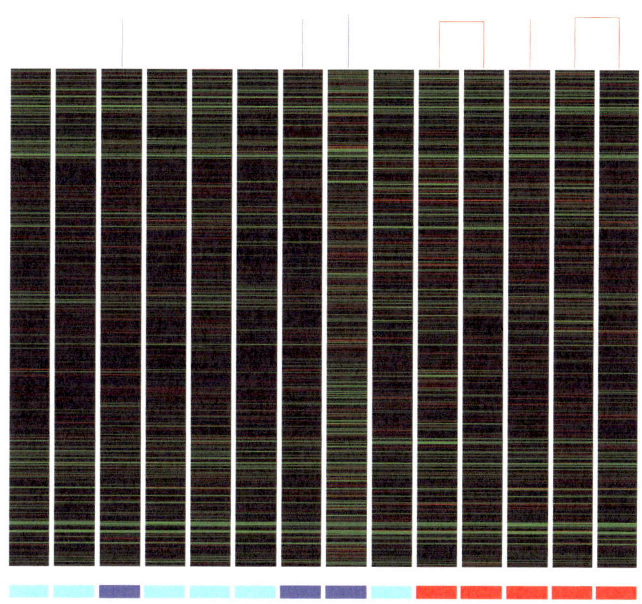

Fig. 3b. Hierarchical clustering analysis (condition tree) of the 14 endometrial samples, displayed as a heat map. Colour code: see legend figure 3a.

3.4 Pathway and network analysis

The list of significantly differentially expressed probe sets (or genes) was further studied with Ingenuity to find the associated canonical pathways and to discover networks between the genes that can be formed based on the available literature. Biological functions that were most significant to the dataset were assigned. In total, 41 networks were derived from the gene list, from which 30 were made up of at least 13 focus molecules (Figure 4).

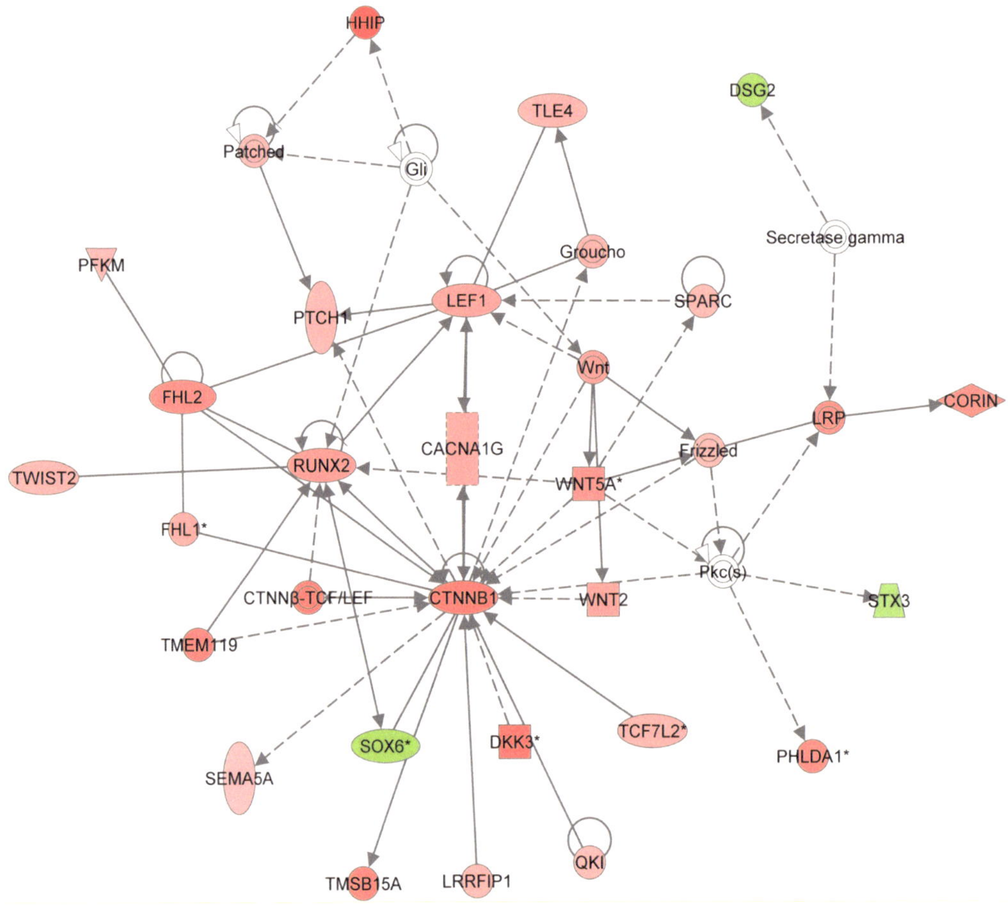

Fig. 4. Network formed on the basis of the literature findings in the Ingenuity database. Upregulated genes from our dataset are coloured red, downregulated genes are coloured green. The shape of the nodes represents the type of molecule (for example enzyme, transcription regulator, group or complex). The lines represent the relationships between the genes (direct or indirect interaction).

The functional analysis identified the biological functions that were most significant to the data set. The top functions were cancer, cellular growth and proliferation, genetic disorders, cellular movement and development and reproductive system diseases (Figure 5).

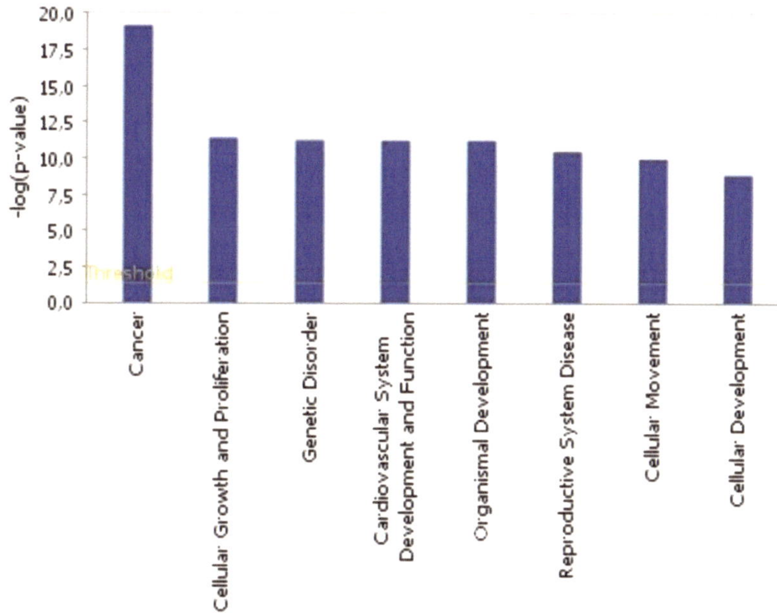

Fig. 5. Overview of the most relevant biological functions or diseases.

Pathway analysis was performed as well (Figure 6). A significant canonical pathway associated with both SOX family members and DKK family members from our data set was the Wnt/ β catenin signalling pathway (Figure 7). This pathway is well known for its role in the reproductive system.

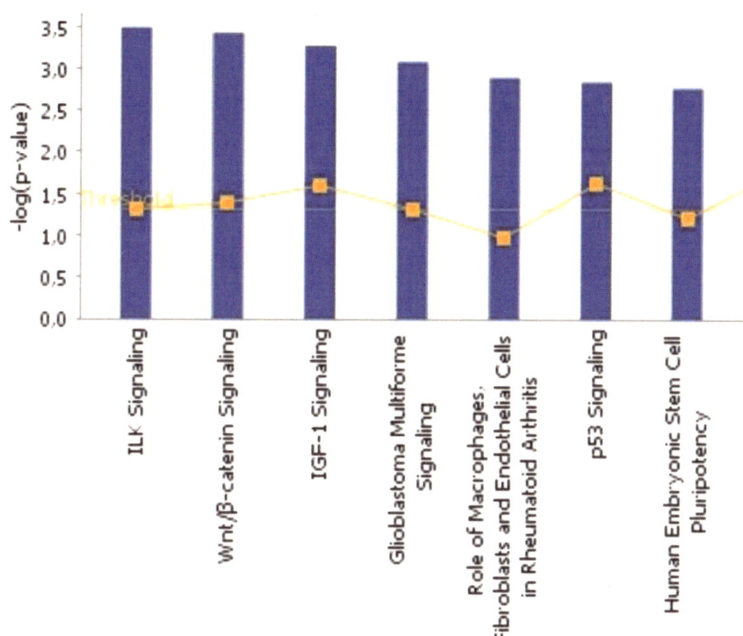

Fig. 6. Overview of the most relevant canonical pathways associated with the data set.

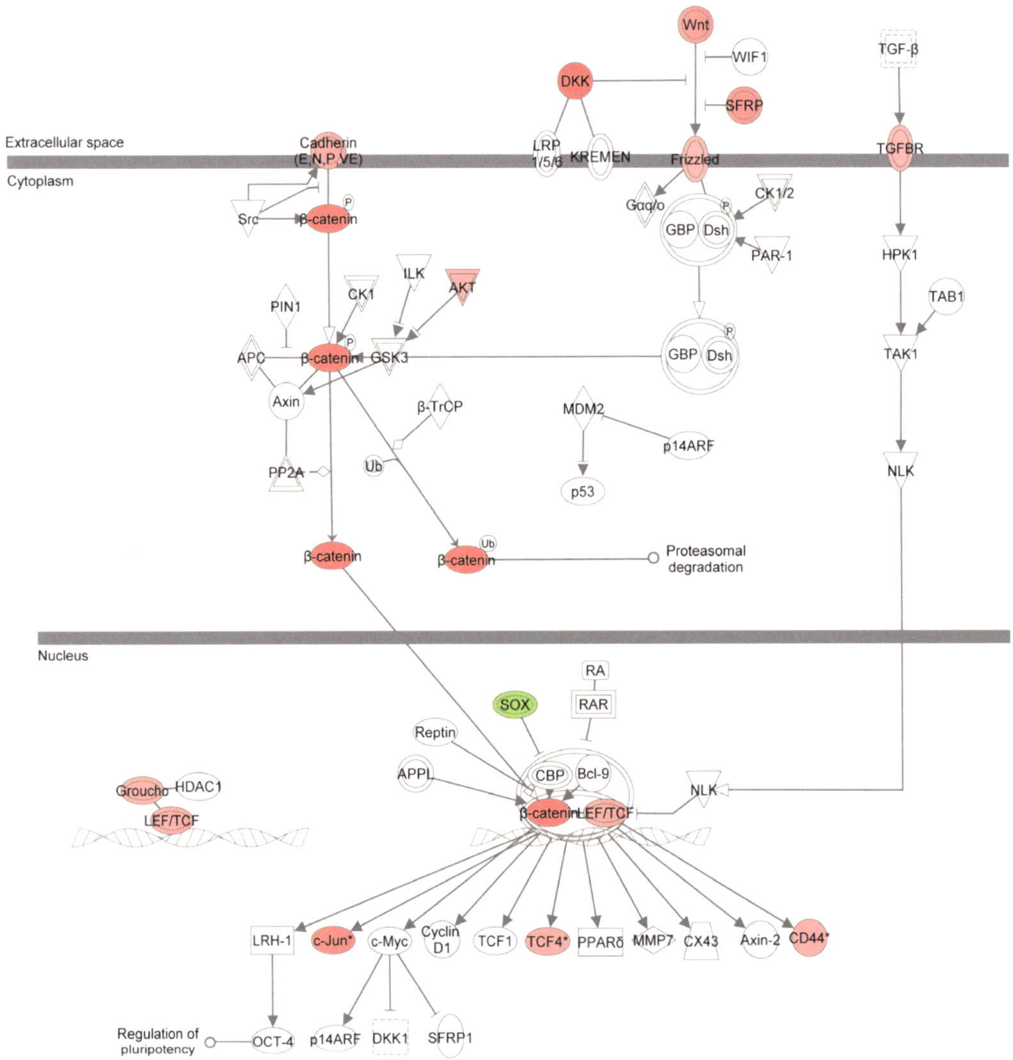

Fig. 7. Wnt/β catenin signalling pathway, in which the DKK (Dickkopf) molecules are upregulated (coloured red) and the SOX family members are downregulated (coloured green), according to our data set.

4. Discussion

Some patients undergoing a stimulated IVF protocol experience premature progesterone elevation towards the end of the follicular phase. Currently, there is an ongoing debate (Van Vaerenbergh et al., 2011 Hum Rep; Al-Azemi et al., submitted to Hum Rep Update) about the aetiology of this premature progesterone rise. It is hypothesized this is due to the high response of the ovary to the stimulation protocol and is associated with lower clinical pregnancy rates (Kyrou et al., 2009: Papanikolaou et al., 2009). In other recent studies, the effect of higher progesterone levels on the endometrial receptivity has been studied as well on the RNA level (Labarta et al., 2011), and even on the microRNA level (Li et al., 2011).

In our study, several groups of patients with premature P rise were compared according to their serum P concentration on the day of hCG administration and in relationship with their gene expression profile on the day of oocyte retrieval. Several genes were selected out of the list of genes which were significantly differentially regulated between the groups with $1 \leq P \leq 1.5$ ng/ml and $P > 1.5$ ng/ml and confirmed with quantitative real-time PCR. The selection of genes occurred according to the criteria described above.

Some of the selected genes were already known for their role(s) in reproductive processes.

During each menstrual cycle, an extensive tissue remodelling process takes place. In the mammalian ovary, proteases are also required for remodelling of the extracellular matrix during follicular growth, breakdown of the follicular wall during ovulation, luteal formation and regression (Curry and Osteen, 2003; Ny et al., 2002). Up to date, several proteases have been implicated in the degradation of the extracellular matrix in the ovary as well as in the endometrium, such as MMPs (matrix metalloproteinases)/TIMPs (Tissue Inhibitor of Metalloproteinases) and ADAMTSs (A Disintegrin And Metalloproteinase with Thrombospondin Motifs).

Protease, serine 23 or PRSS23 is an extracellular serine protease expressed in the mouse ovary and may play a role in follicular development in the mouse. PRSS23 is highly expressed in atretic follicles and in the ovarian stroma and thecal layers just before ovulation. Its dynamic expression pattern suggests that PRSS23 is involved in different tissue remodelling processes in the ovary, possibly by allowing extracellular matrix degradation and/or regulating growth factor availability (Miyakoshi et al., 2006; Wahlberg et al., 2008).

THSD4 (thrombospondin, type I, domain containing 4) is an ADAMTS-like protein and has been described in human endometrium in a stimulated cycle in another study performed in the Centre for Reproductive Medicine (Blockeel et al., 2011).

The interleukin 17 receptor B (IL17RB or IL17BR) is an estrogen-regulated gene (Wang et al., 2007) and found to be a prognostic marker, together with homeobox 13 expression, for breast cancer (Jerevall et al., 2008; Ma et al., 2008). In general, interleukins, chemokines, cytokines and other immunological molecules are known to play a major role during implantation. (Lindhard et al., 2002).

Another protease is PAPP-A or IGFBP4 (insulin-like growth factor-binding protein-4), a metalloproteinase from the metzincin superfamily (Boldt and Conover, 2007; Conover et al., 2004; Ohnishi et al., 2005; Overgaard et al., 1999). This family also includes the astacins, serralysins, adamalysins (ADAMTS) and the matrix metalloproteinases (MMP) (Huxley-Jones et al., 2007; Reiss et al., 2006). PAPP-A acts as a protease for IGFBP4 and in this way helps releasing IGF (insulin-like growth factor). IGF-II has a major role in implantation and trophoblast invasion (Giudice et al., 2002). Insuline-like growth factors can bind to six IGF-binding proteins, IGFBP1-6, which are able to modulate IGF actions in various ways (Suzuki et al., 2006). PAPP-A is produced by the trophoblasts and also known as a sensitive marker for adverse pregnancy outcome in the first trimester (Suzuki et al., 2006). Human decidualized endometrial stromal cells secrete PAPP-A as well (Giudice et al., 2002).

The Wnt/β-catenin signalling pathway has been described before in different implantation-related and endometrial receptivity studies (Tulac et al., 2003; Van Vaerenbergh et al., 2009).

Furthermore, another member of the Dickkopf family, DKK1, has been observed in the mid-secretory phase (LH+7) of a natural cycle in several endometrial receptivity gene expression studies (Carson et al., 2002; Haouzi et al., 2009; Riesewijk et al., 2003; Talbi et al., 2006).

Previous studies (Kolibianakis et al., 2002; Ubaldi et al., 1997) with endometrial biopsies on the day of oocyte retrieval and following embryo transfer demonstrated that an endometrial advancement of more than 3 days never resulted in a clinical pregnancy. From an earlier study in our group (Van Vaerenbergh et al., 2009), these findings were confirmed on the gene expression level with microarrays. It was found that endometrial samples taken on the day of oocyte retrieval from patients in a GnRH antagonist/ rec-FSH stimulation protocol for IVF with embryo transfer all showed an advanced endometrial maturation and that the samples with an advanced endometrium of more than 3 days clustered together in a separate molecular profile.

In this study, no clinical pregnancies were seen when the P concentration was higher than 1.5 ng/ml. All four clinical pregnancies ensued in patients from groups with $P \leq 0.9$ ng/ml and with $1 \leq P \leq 1.5$ ng/ml.

A large group of significantly differentially expressed probe sets was observed between the group with progesterone levels between 1 and 1.5 ng/ml ($1 \leq P \leq 1.5$ ng/ml) and the group with progesterone levels above 1.5 ng/ml. Moreover, hierarchical clustering analysis and principal component analysis showed a separate cluster for patients in the group with progesterone concentrations above 1.5 ng/ml. The clustering pattern possibly also reflects the state of endometrial maturation of the biopsy, as one sample dated as +day 4, is more closely situated near the cluster from the group with the highest progesterone concentrations. Although, there is a trend noticeable that patients with premature progesterone rise on the day of hCG administration have a morphological advanced secretory endometrium, this is not always true. In the current study, it can be demonstrated from the clustering analyses and the available histological dating results that the elevation of progesterone levels in the follicular phase seems somehow related to the endometrial maturation state, although predicting the histological date of the endometrial biopsy is not possible.

5. Conclusion

This is the first study to investigate the endometrial gene expression on the day of oocyte retrieval in stimulated cycles for IVF with embryo transfer, according to the concentration of progesterone on the day of hCG administration.

In conclusion, the early elevation of progesterone on the day of hCG administration seems to have an instant effect on the endometrial gene expression, as shown by a biopsy sample taken only 36 hours later, on the day of oocyte retrieval. The threshold for P concentration with a distinct different molecular profile was found at 1.5 ng/ml.

These significant changes observed at the gene expression level may explain the impairment of endometrial receptivity in the presence of elevated progesterone, reflected in the lower clinical pregnancy rates as reported in recent publications (Bosch et al., 2003; 2010; Kolibianakis et al., 2011).

6. Acknowledgment

This study was originally published in Reproductive Biomedicine Online (Van Vaerenbergh et al., 2011).

Furthermore, we would like to thank the Fonds Wetenschappelijk Onderzoek - Vlaanderen (FWO) for its financial support with grant G031707N (FWO AL405) during this study.

7. References

Al-Azemi M, Kyrou D, Kolibianakis EM, Humaidan P, Van Vaerenbergh I, Devroey P, Fatemi HM. Elevated Progesterone during Ovarian Stimulation for In-Vitro Fertilization. SUBMITTED

Blockeel C, Van Vaerenbergh I, Fatemi HM, Van Lommel L, Devroey P, Bourgain C. Gene expression profile in the endometrium on the day of oocyte retrieval after ovarian stimulation with low-dose hCG in the follicular phase. Mol Hum Reprod, 2011;17(1):33-41.

Boldt HB, Conover CA. Pregnancy-associated plasma protein-A (PAPP-A): a local regulator of IGF bioavailability through cleavage of IGFBPs. Growth Horm IGF Res, 2007;17(1):10-8.

Bosch E, Valencia I, Escudero E, Crespo J, Simon C, Remohi J, Pellicer A. Premature luteinisation during gonadotropin-releasing hormone antagonist cycles and its relationship with in vitro fertilization outcome. Fertil Steril, 2003;80(6):1444-9.

Bosch E, Labarta E, Crespo J, Simon C, Remohi J, Jenkins J, Pellicer A. Circulating progesterone levels and ongoing pregnancy rates in controlled ovarian stimulation cycles for in vitro fertilization: analysis of over 4000 cycles. Hum Reprod, 2010;25(8):2092-100.

Carson DD, Lagow E, Thathiah A, Al-Shami R, Farach-Carson MC, Vernon M, Yuan L, Fritz MA, Lessey B. Changes in gene expression during the early to mid-luteal (receptive phase) transition in human endometrium detected by high-density microarray screening. Mol Hum Reprod, 2002;8(9):871-9.

Conover CA, Bale LK, Overgaard MT, Johnstone EW, Laursen UH, Füchtbauer EM, Oxvig C, van Deursen J. Metalloproteinase pregnancy-associated plasma protein A is a criticalgrowth regulatory factor during fetal development. Development, 2004;131(5):1187-94.

Curry TE Jr, Osteen KG. The matrix metalloproteinase system: changes, regulation, and impact throughout the ovarian and uterine reproductive cycle. Endocr Rev, 2003;24(4):428–465.

Edelstein MC, Seltman HJ, Cox BJ, Robinson SM, Shaw RA, Muasher SJ. Progesterone levels on the day of human chorionic gonadotropin administration in cycles with gonadotropin-releasing hormone agonist suppression are not predictive of pregnancy outcome. Fertil Steril 1990;54:853-857.

Eisen MB, Spellman PT, Brown PO, Botstein D. Cluster analysis and display of genomewide expression patterns. Proc Natl Acad Sci USA, 1998;95(25):14863–14868.

Giudice LC, Conover CA, Bale L, Faessen GH, Ilg K, Sun I, Imani B, Suen LF, Irwin JC, Christiansen M, Overgaard MT, Oxvig C. Identification and regulation of the IGFBP-4 protease and its physiological inhibitor in human trophoblasts and endometrial stroma: evidence for paracrine regulation of IGF-II bioavailability in the placental bed during human implantation. J Clin Endocrinol Metab, 2002;87(5):2359-2366.

Givens CR, Schriock ED, Dandekar PV, Martin MC. Elevated serum progesterone levels on the day of human chorionic gonadotropin administration do not predict outcome in assisted reproduction cycles. Fertil Steril 1994; 62:1011-1017.

Haouzi D, Mahmoud K, Fourar M, Bendhaou K, Dechaud H, De Vos J, Rème T, Dewailly D, Hamamah S. Identification of new biomarkers of human endometrial receptivity in the natural cycle. Hum Reprod. 2009 ;24(1):198-205.

Hofmann GE, Bentzien F, Bergh PA, Garrisi GJ, Williams MC, Guzman I, Navot D. Premature luteinization in controlled ovarian hyperstimulation has no adverse effect on oocyte and embryo quality. Fertil Steril, 1993;60(4):675-9.

Huxley-Jones J, Clarke TK, Beck C, Toubaris G, Robertson DL, Boot-Handford RP. The evolution of the vertebrate metzincins; insights from Ciona intestinalis and Danio rerio. BMC Evol Biol, 2007;17(7):63.

Jerevall PL, Brommesson S, Strand C, Gruvberger-Saal S, Malmström P, Nordenskjöld B, Wingren S, Söderkvist P, Fernö M, Stål O. Exploring the two-gene ratio in breast cancer—independent roles for HOXB13 and IL17BR in prediction of clinical outcome. Breast Cancer Res Treat, 2008;107(2):225-34.

Kolibianakis EM, Venetis CA, Bontis J, Tarlatzis BC. Significantly Lower Pregnancy Rates in the Presence of Progesterone Elevation in Patients Treated with GnRH Antagonists and Gonadotrophins: A Systematic Review and Meta-Analysis. Curr Pharm Biotechnol. 2011 Jun 9. [Epub ahead of print]

Kolibianakis E, Bourgain C, Albano C, Osmanagaoglu K, Smitz J, Van Steirteghem A, Devroey P. Effect of ovarian stimulation with recombinant follicle-stimulating hormone, gonadotropin releasing hormone antagonists, and human chorionic gonadotropin on endometrial maturation on the day of oocyte pick-up. Fertil Steril, 2002;78(5):1025–1029.

Kyrou D, Popovic-Todorovic B, Fatemi HM, Bourgain C, Haentjens P, Van Landuyt L, Devroey P. Does the estradiol level on the day of human chorionic gonadotrophin administration have an impact on pregnancy rates in patients treated with rec-FSH/GnRH antagonist? Hum Reprod, 2009;24(11):2902-9.

Labarta E, Martínez-Conejero JA, Alamá P, Horcajadas JA, Pellicer A, Simón C, Bosch E. Endometrial receptivity is affected in women with high circulating progesterone levels at the end of the follicular phase: a functional genomics analysis. Hum Reprod. 2011 Jul;26(7):1813-25.

Lindhard A, Bentin-Ley U, Ravn V, Islin H, Hviid T, Rex S, Bangsbøll S, Sørensen S. Biochemical evaluation of endometrial function at the time of implantation. Fertil Steril 2002;78(2):221-33.

Li R, Qiao J, Wang L, Li L, Zhen X, Liu P, Zheng X. MicroRNA array and microarray evaluation of endometrial receptivity in patients with high serum progesterone levels on the day of hCG administration. Reproductive Biology and Endocrinology 2011, 9:29

Ma XJ, Salunga R, Dahiya S, Wang W, Carney E, Durbecq V, Harris A, Goss P, Sotiriou C, Erlander M, Sgroi D. A five-gene molecular grade index and HOXB13:IL17BR are complementary prognostic factors in early stage breast cancer. Clin Cancer Res, 2008;14(9):2601-8.

Miyakoshi K, Murphy MJ, Yeoman RR, Mitra S, Dubay CJ, Hennebold JD. The identification of novel ovarian proteases through the use of genomic and bioinformatics methodologies. Biol Reprod, 2006;75(6):823-835.

Noyes RW, Hertig AT, Rock J. Dating the endometrial biopsy. Fertil Steril, 1950;1:3-25.

Ny T, Wahlberg P, Brändström IJ. Matrix remodeling in the ovary: regulation and functional role of the plasminogen activator and matrix metalloproteinase systems. Mol Cell Endocrinol, 2002;187(1-2):29-38.

Ohnishi J, Ohnishi E, Shibuya H, Takahashi T. Functions for proteinases in the ovulatory process. Biochimica et Biophysica Acta, 2005;1751(1):95-109.

Overgaard MT, Oxvig C, Christiansen M, Lawrence JB, Conover CA, Gleich GJ, Sottrup-Jensen L, Haaning J. Messenger ribonucleic acid levels of pregnancy associated plasma protein-A and the proform of eosinophil major basic protein: expression in human reproductive and nonreproductive tissues. Biol Reprod, 1999;61(4):1083-1089.

Papanikolaou EG, Kolibianakis EM, Pozzobon C, Tank P, Tournaye H, Bourgain C, Van Steirteghem A, Devroey P. Progesterone rise on the day of human chorionic gonadotropin administration impairs pregnancy outcome in day 3 single-embryo transfer, while has no effect on day 5 single blastocyst transfer. Fertil Steril, 2009;91(3):949-952.

Reiss K, Ludwig A, Saftig P. Breaking up the tie: disintegrin-like metalloproteinases as regulators of cell migration in inflammation and invasion. Pharmacol Ther, 2006;111(3):985-1006.

Riesewijk A, Martín J, van Os R, Horcajadas JA, Polman J, Pellicer A, Mosselman S, Simon C. Gene expression profiling of human endometrial receptivity on days LH+2 versus LH+7 by microarray technology. Mol Hum Reprod, 2003;9(5):253-64.

Rotterdam ESHRE/ASRM-Sponsored PCOS Consensus Workshop Group. Revised 2003 consensus on diagnostic criteria and long-term health risks related to polycystic ovary syndrome. Fertil Steril, 2004;81(1):19–25.

Silverberg KM, Burns WN, Olive DL, Riehl RM, Schenken RS. Serum progesterone levels predict success of in vitro fertilization/embryo transfer in patients stimulated with leuprolide acetate and human menopausal gonadotropins. J Clin Endocrinol Metab 1991;73:797-803.

Silverberg KM, Martin M, Olive DL, Burns WN, Schenken RS. Elevated serum progesterone levels on the day of human chorionic gonadotropin administration in in vitro fertilization cycles do not adversely affect embryo quality. Fertil Steril 1994;61:508-513.

Suzuki K, Sata F, Yamada H, Saijo Y, Tsuruga N, Minakami H, Kishi R. Pregnancyassociated plasma protein-A polymorphism and the risk of recurrent pregnancy loss. J Reprod Immunol, 2006;70(1-2):99-108.

Talbi S, Hamilton AE, Vo KC, Tulac S, Overgaard MT, Dosiou C, Le Shay N, Nezhat CN, Kempson R, Lessey BA, Nayak NR, Giudice LC. Molecular phenotyping of human endometrium distinguishes menstrual cycle phases and underlying biological processes in normo-ovulatory women. Endocrinology, 2006;147(3):1097-121.

Tulac S, Nayak NR, Kao LC, Van Waes M, Huang J, Lobo S, Germeyer A, Lessey BA, Taylor RN, Suchanek E, Giudice LC. Identification, characterization, and regulation of the canonical Wnt signaling pathway in human endometrium. J Clin Endocrinol Metab, 2003;88(8):3860–3866.

Ubaldi F, Albano C, Peukert M, Riethmuller-Winzen H, Camus M, Smitz J, Van Steirteghem A, Devroey P. Subtle progesterone rise after administration of the gonadotrophin-releasing hormone antagonist cetrorelix in intracytoplasmic sperm injection cycles. Hum Reprod 1996;11:1405-1407.

Ubaldi F, Bourgain C, Tournaye H, Smitz J, Van Steirteghem A, Devroey P. Endometrial evaluation by aspiration biopsy on the day of oocyte retrieval in the embryo transfer cycles in patients with serum progesterone rise during the follicular phase. Fertil Steril, 1997;67(3):521–526.

Van Landuyt L, De Vos A, Joris H, Verheyen G, Devroey P, Van Steirteghem A. Blastocyst formation in in vitro fertilization versus intracytoplasmic sperm injection cycles: influence of the fertilization procedure. Fertil Steril 2005;83:1397-1403.

Van Vaerenbergh I, Fatemi HM, Blockeel C, Van Lommel L, In't Veld P, Schuit F, Kolibianakis EM, Devroey P, Bourgain C. Progesterone rise on hCG day in GnRH antagonist/rec-FSH stimulated cycles affects endometrial gene expression. RBM Online, 2011;22(3):263-271.

Van Vaerenbergh I, Fatemi HM and Bourgain C. Premature progesterone rise and gene expression. Hum Reprod. 2011 Oct;26(10):2913.

Van Vaerenbergh I, Van Lommel L, Ghislain V, In't Veld P, Schuit F, Fatemi HM, Devroey P, Bourgain C. In GnRH antagonist/rec-FSH stimulated cycles, advanced endometrial maturation on the day of oocyte retrieval correlates with altered gene expression. Hum Reprod, 2009;24(5):1085-1091.

Venetis CA, Kolibianakis EM, Papanikolaou E, Bontis J, Devroey P, Tarlatzis BC. Is progesterone elevation on the day of human chorionic gonadotrophin administration associated with the propability of pregnancy in in vitro fertilization? A systematic review and meta-analysis. Hum Reprod Update, 2007;13(4):343-355.

Wahlberg P, Nylander A, Ahlskog N, Liu K, Ny T. Expression and localization of the serine proteases high-temperature requirement factor A1, serine protease 23, and serine protease 35 in the mouse ovary. Endocrinology, 2008;149(10):5070-5077.

Wang H, Xie H, Sun X, Tranguch S, Zhang H, Jia X, Wang D, Das SK, Desvergne B, Wahli W, DuBois RN, Dey SK. Stage-specific integration of maternal and embryonic PPARdelta signaling is critical to pregnancy success. J Biol Chem, 2007;282(52):37770–82.

Zegers-Hochschild F, Adamson GD, de Mouzon J, Ishihara O, Mansour R, Nygren K, Sullivan E, van der Poel S; International Committee for Monitoring Assisted Reproductive Technology; World Health Organization. The International Committee for Monitoring Assisted Reproductive Technology (ICMART) and the World Health Organization (WHO) Revised Glossary on ART Terminology, 2009. Hum Reprod 2009;24(11):2683-2687.

3

The Role of Ultrasound in the Evaluation of Endometrial Receptivity Following Assisted Reproductive Treatments

Mitko Ivanovski
St. Lazar Hospital, Skopje
Macedonia

1. Introduction

Improvements in in vitro fertilization (IVF) and embryo transfer (ET) have resulted from evaluating each step of the process, analyzing effects of different techniques, then assessing outcomes to select the best method, whether related to preparation of the patient, choice of stimulation protocol, culture technique, embryo selection, mechanics of transfer, or posttransfer management. Despite numerous developments in assisted reproduction, the clinical pregnancy rate (CPR) in IVF and intracytoplasmatic sperm injection (ICSI) remains low. It has been estimated that up to 85% of the embryos replaced into the uterine cavity fail to implant (Edwards RG, 1995). The cause of this low CPR may reside in the technique of embryo transfer, the endometrial receptivity, or the capacity of the embryo to properly invade the endometrium.

Endometrial receptivity is defined as a temporary unique sequence of factors that make the endometrium receptive to the embryonic implantation. It is the window of time when the uterine environment is conductive to blastocyst acceptance and subsequent implantation. The process of implantation may be separated into a series of developmental phases starting with the blastocyst hatching and attachment to the endometrium and culminating in the formation of the placenta. The steps start with apposition, and progress through adhesion, penetration and invasion. Evaluation of endometrial receptivity remains a challenge in clinical practice.

Ultrasonography has an increasingly important role in the evaluation and treatment of infertility patients, being an efficient and cost-effective modality for studying the female reproductive organs and for monitoring functional changes during spontaneous and induced cycles (Blumenfeld et al., 1990; Goldberg et al., 1991).

Two-dimensional (2D) ultrasound imagining is limited by the movement of the transvaginal transducer in the narrow space of vagina. Therefore, it allows presentation of two planes: sagital and transverse. Real time ultrasonography allows us the study of two main implantation markers: endometrial thickness and endometrial morphological patterns. (Merce, 2002). Pulsed and color Doppler assessment is applied to the study of different variables of uterine and endometrial/subendometrial perfusion that are also used as receptivity factors (Fanchin, 2001).

Three - dimensional (3D) sonography permits multiplanar display of all three sections: coronal, sagittal and transverse. The three-dimensional (3D) approach to assessing uterine receptivity, which considers endometrial thickness as well as volume, uterine artery Doppler and also endometrial tissue vascularization itself, might lead to a better understanding of this very specific and crucial endometrial preparation for implantation. The 3D technique allows reliable quantification of the two crucial phenomena—tissue remodeling pattern and tissue associated angiogenic dynamics—with quantification of the sub-endometrial vascular flow index.

The Embryo transfer (ET) procedure is the final important step in IVF process. It is a critically important procedure. No matter how good the IVF laboratory culture environment is, the physician can ruin everything with a carelessly performed embryo transfer. The entire IVF cycle depends on delicate placement of the embryos at the proper location of the endometrial cavity - with minimal trauma and manipulation. It has been suggested that ultrasound-guided ET (2D end 3/4D) facilitates ET and improves pregnancy rates, because it is thought that visualization of the cavity and the embryo deposition point have an advantage in comparison with blind ET technique.

2. Assessment of the endometrium implantation markers with ultrasound

Assessment of the endometrium has become a standard procedure during the diagnostic workup and treatment of infertility. Ultrasound sees the endometrium as a single thin line immediately after menstruation. This then expands under the influence of oestrogen in the follicular phase of the cycle to the typical trilaminar hypoechoic appearance. After ovulation there is little increase in size. The change to a secretory state is characterized by increasing echogenicity beginning at the periphery of the endometrium and progressing towards the midline over a period of 24–48 h. The mature luteal endometrium appears homogenous and hyperechoic compared with the myometrium.

Real time ultrasonography allows us the study of three main possible implantation markers: endometrial thickness, endometrial volume and endometrial morphological patterns.

2.1 Endometrial thickness

Endometrial thickness is defined as the maximal distance between the echogenic interfaces of the myometrium and the endometrium, measured in the plane through the central longitudinal axis of the uterus.

Dynamic change in endometrial thickness in assisted conception cycles was first described by Rabinowitz et al. (1986). Using transvaginal scanning, Gonen et al.(1989) suggested that endometrial thickness, on the day before oocyte recovery, was significantly greater in pregnant than in non-pregnant women, and postulated that it may predict the likelihood of implantation. In IVF stimulated cycles, the endometrium increases 1.9 mm between days 7 and 9 of the stimulation treatment, 0.9 mm between days 9 and 11 and 0.6 mm between the latter and the day of hCG administration (Bassil et al.,2001). Significant differences have not been observed in endometrial thickness between hCG day and the day of embryo transfer (Khalifa et al., 1992), which clearly has practical implications to choose the timing for the measurement. In the conception cycles there is an accelerated increase in the endometrial thickness during the luteal phase that reaches significant differences regarding to that in non-conception cycles 14 days after the day of oocyte retrieval (Leibovitz et al., 1999; Rhabinowitz et al.,1986).

As an implantation marker, endometrial thickness is characterized by its significant sensitivity (95-100%), but also shows a high number of false positives (78-97%) (Friedler et al., 1996), therefore, the main advantage is a high negative predictive value (87-100%). The main advantage of measuring endometrial thickness lies in its high negative predictive value in cases where there is minimal endometrial thickness. In IVF cycles, Khalifa et al. (1992) reported a minimal endometrial thickness of 7 mm to be accepted as a reliable sign of sub-optimal implantation potential. Although it is possible to achieve pregnancies with a thin endometrium (Remohi et al., 1997; Sundstrom 1998), this is always a bad predictive factor that requires further study of the endometrium (Noyes et al.,2001). It has also been reported that implantation , pregnancy and miscarriage rates are negatively affected by the endometrium being thicker than 14mm (Dickey at al., 1992; Noyes et al.,2001; Remohi et al.,1997; Weisman et al.,1999), although data from recent studies do not support this finding (Krampl and Feichtinger ,1993; Dietterich et al.,2002; Zhang et al.,2005). There is a positive correlation between increased endometrial thickness and pregnancy rates and further explained that this effect is dependent on the age of the patient, duration of stimulation, and embryo quality (Rabinowitz et al., 1986; Zhang et al., 2005). Contrary to these data, other studies show that measurement of endometrial thickness had no predictive value for pregnancy in ART (Fleischer et al., 1986; Glissant et al., 1985; Ivanovski et al., 2007a; Li et al., 1992; Welker et al., 1989).

Amir et al. (2007) reported that the possibility of a thick endometrium in IVF administered women over the age of 40 is less than that of the younger patient group; however, he also reported that pregnancy rate increases in the presence of thick endometrium.

Freidler et al. (1996) reviewed 2665 assisted conception cycles from 25 reports. Eight reports found that the difference in the mean endometrial thickness of conception and non-conception cycles was statistically significant, while 17 reports found no significant difference. They concluded that results from various trials are conflicting and that insufficient data exist describing a linear correlation between endometrial thickness and the probability of conception. There is not enough data to demonstrate if a linear relationship exists between endometrial thickness and the probability of pregnancy after an ART (Friedler et al., 1996).

2.2 Endometrial volume

Transvaginal 2D ultrasonography is an ideal non-invasive method for assessment of endometrium, but lacks specificity (Friedler et al., 1996). The use of 3 D ultrasonography to examine the uterine cavity in detail and reconstruct the images of the uterus surpasses the diagnostic potential of Two Dimensional (2D) ultrasound (Jurkovic et al., 1995; Lev-Toaff et al., 2001). Using two dimensional transvaginal ultrasound to measure endometrial thickness does not include the total volume of the endometrium (Friedler et al., 1996). Several studies have confirmed a high degree of reproducibility and accuracy of endometrial volume estimation using 3D ultrasound (Lee et al., 1997; Yaman et al., 2000).

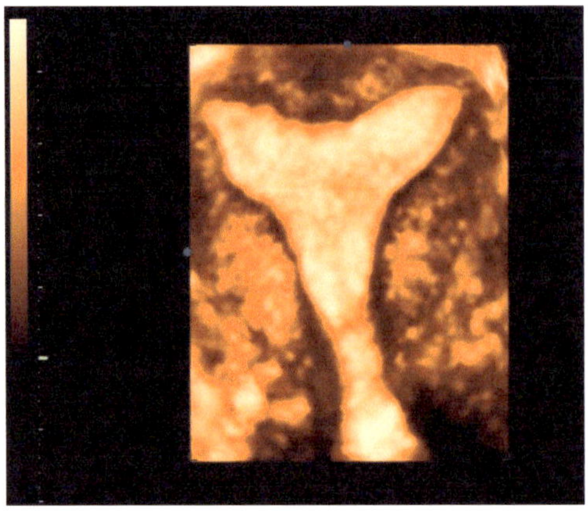

Photo 1. 3D Ultrasound of uterus and endometrium

3D US images can be obtained by two methods: freehand and automated. The freehand method requires manual movement of the transducer through the region of interest. The automated method acquires the images using dedicated 3D transducers. The digitally stored volume data can be manipulated and presented in various displays: multiplanar display, "niche" mode or surface rendering mode (Alcasar, 2006). Probably, the most used and useful display is multiplanar display, which simultaneously shows three perpendicular planes (axial, sagital and coronal), allowing navigation through these three planes with the possibility of switch over any desired plane. Another important ability of 3D US is volume calculation, even in irregularly shaped structures, using the Virtual Organ Computer-aided AnaLysis (VOCAL).

This method has been demonstrated to be more accurate than 2D-volume estimation, with an error estimation of 7% for 3D US as compared of 22% for 2D US (Yaman et al., 2003)]. Other investigators described a mean absolute error rate of 12.6% for two dimensional volume measurements, while the absolute error rate for 3D volume measurement was only 6.4% (Riccabona et al., 1996).

During spontaneous menstrual cycles endometrial volume increased significantly during the follicular phase, reaching a plateau around the time of ovulation and remaining relatively stable throughout the luteal phase (Jakubkiene et al., 2006; Reine-Fenning et al., 2004). Parous women showed endometrial volumes significantly larger than nulliparous women (Reine-Fenning et al., 2004).

3D technology has added to daily practice in reproduction the use of endometrial volume as an implantation marker (Merce, 2004). Schild at al. (1999) was the first to correlate endometrial volume on the day of oocyte retrieval and pregnancy rate in an IVF program. They found that endometrial volume failed to predict outcome of IVF and that estradiol levels did not correlate with endometrial volume. Almost simultaneously, Raga et al. (1999) reported on 72 patients who underwent IVF cycle, using the same technique that Schild et al. (1999) for calculating endometrial volume but ultrasound examination was performed on the day of embryo transfer. These authors found that pregnancy rate was significantly lower (15%) if endometrial volume was < 2 ml than if it was > 2 ml (34.5%). No pregnancy was achieved with endometrial volume below 1 ml. Yaman et al.(2000) reported subsequently in

65 patients undergoing IVF program [47]. They found that endometrial volume did not differ significantly in women that became pregnant from those who did not. No pregnancy occurred of endometrial volume was < 2.5 ml. Zollner et al.(2003) evaluated endometrial volume in 125 women undergoing IVF. They found that pregnancy rate was lower in patients with endometrial volume < 2.5 ml (9.4%) compared with those with endometrial volume ≥2.5 ml (35%).

All studies more recently published have not demonstrated that endometrial volume is predictive for pregnancy after IVF program (Jarvela et al., 2005; Kupesic et al., 2001; Ng et al., 2006; Schild et al., 2000; Wu et al., 2003). This could be explained by methodological differences in volume calculation.

In our study clear morphology of the endometrium was obtained in 106 patients using 3D transvaginal ultrasound at the time of embryo transfer. The mean endometrial volume (±2SD) vas 3.27±0.69 (range 1.7 - 7.9). Women were divided into three groups depending on the endometrial volume data: group 1: < 2ml; group 2 : 2-5 ml; group 3 ; > 5 ml respectively. No differences in age, number of days of ovarian stimulation, total , number of oocyte retrieved, and number of good quality embryios were found between these groups (table 1). Patients with an andometrial volume < 2ml (group1) had significantly (p<0.05) lower pregnancy and implantation rates as compared with the groups of women with 2-5 ml (group 2) and >5ml (group 3) endometrial volume. Moreover, no differences were observed between the latter two groups.

Parameter	**Group1: < 2 ml**	**Group 2: 2-5 ml**	**Group 3: > 5 ml**	**p**
Cycles No	30	42	36	
Age (years)	35±0.9	34±0.8	32±0.5	NS
Treatment (days)	9.6±0.3	9.3±0.49	9.1±0.36	NS
Oocytes retrieved No	9±2.9	11±2.1	12±2.7	NS
No embryo transfer	2.4±0.5	2.2±0.3	25±0.6	NS
No of pregnancies	5 (16.6%)	14 (33%)	13 (36%)	P<0.05

Table 1. Patients grouped according to endometrial volume on the day of embryo transfer

An endometrial volume of 2.5 ml on the day of embryo transfer has been proposed as a reliable threshold value to predict pregnancy after embryo transfer in IVF/ICSI cycles. However, again these findings lacked of specificity.

2.3 Endometrial pattern

Endometrial pattern is defined as the relative echogenicity of the endometrium and the adjacent myometrium as demonstrated on a longitudinal ultrasound scan. During the proliferative phase of the menstrual cycle the endometrium achieves a "triple line" morphology. In principle, the central echogenic line represents the uterine cavity; the outer lines represent the basal layer of the endometrium, or the interface between the endometrium and myometrium. The relatively hypo-echogenic regions between two outer lines and the central line may represent the functional layer of endometrium (Forest et al.,

1988). During the secretory phase of the menstrual cycle, the endometrium acquires a hyperechogenic morphology that is due to stromal edema, spirilization and secretion of the endometrial glands caused by the action of progesterone (Bassil et al., 2001; Fanchin et al., 2000; Fanchin et al., 2001; Leibovitz et al., 1999). However, since a correlation between echogenicity and progesterone has not been demonstrated (Bakos et al., 1993; Khalife et al., 1992) other factors such as androgen and gonadotropin effects could explain these changes (De Ziegler and Fancin, 1994; Tang and Gurpide, 1993).

Classification of the types of appearance of the endometrium has been simplified over time. Nowadays, intermediate patterns are often discarded and the endometrium is simply described as multilayered or non-multilayered (Sher et al., 1991; Smith et al., 1984). In a prospective study, Serafimi et al.(1994) found the multilayered pattern to be more predictive of implantation than any other parameter measured. The "triple line" endometrial pattern has high sensitivity (79-100%) but an elevated percentage of false positives (57-91%) also, subsequently it has an additional interest by its high negative predictive value (75-100%). Although achieving a pregnancy with a "non triple-line" pattern is possible, its frequency is low (Tan et al., 2000).

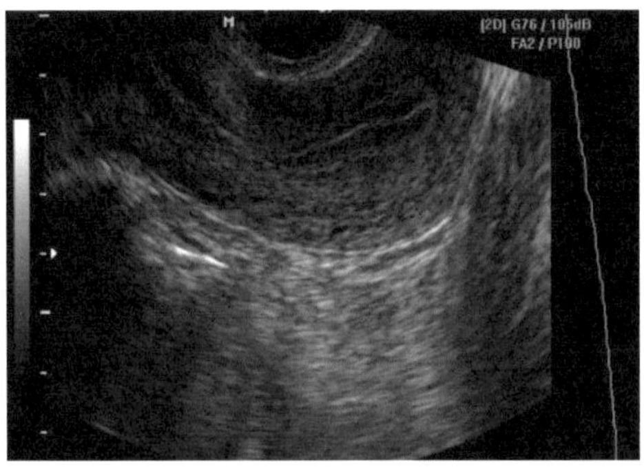

Photo 2. Multilayered endometrium

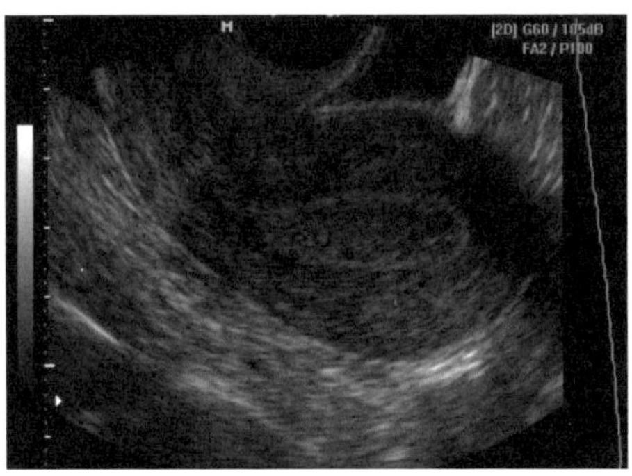

Photo 3. Non multilayered endometrium

The normal luteal endometrial pattern has been also implied as an implantation marker. A non-homogeneous hyperechogenic pattern 3 days after embryo transfer has been associated with lower pregnancy rates (Check et al., 2000). In addition, the midluteal endometrial pattern of women with unexplained infertility is related to the chance of pregnancy. The pregnancy rate is significantly higher when the endometrium displays a homogenous hyperechogenic pattern comparatively with non-homogenous pattern (Check et al., 2003). It is, however, important to emphasize that a poor endometrial pattern does not exclude pregnancy.

Our observation showed that 15(17.65%) patients have homogenous endometrium, and the other 70 (82.35%) have triple line endometrium. There was not statistical significant difference, p>0.05(p=1.00)/ Fisher) according pregnancy rates between both groups of patients (Table 2).

Endometrial pattern	BHCG +	BHCG -	Total
Homogenous	5	10	15
Total %	5.88	11.76	17.65
Triple line	24	46	70
Total %	28.24	54.12	82.35
Total	29	56	85
Total %	34.12	65.88	100

Table 2. Endometrial pattern and pregnancy outcome

The effect of endometrial thickness and hyperechogenic pattern on determining pregnancy outcomes have been presented with various results. Increased endometrial thickness, endometrial pattern, and volume affect IVF outcomes, and this effect is dependent on patient's age, duration of stimulation, and embryo quality (Richter et al., 2007; Zhang et al., 2005). Tsai et al.(2000) reported that in ovulation induction by administering CC and gonadotropin and in IUI cycles, in terms of endometrial parameters, endometrial pattern has a significant effect on pregnancy positive and pregnancy negative patients; however, thickness and vascularity do not change pregnancy results. Fanchin et al. (2000) supported this view and reported that hyperechogenic endometrium deteriorates IVF outcomes.

Kepic et al.(1992) determined that endometrial thickness and pattern, follicle size and estradiol levels correlated to both the likelihood of pregnancy and subsequent outcome. Contrary to these data, other studies found no correlation between endometrial thickness, endometrial pattern and embryo implantation (Fleischer et al., 1986; Friedler et al., 1996; Ivanovski et al., 2007a; Rashidi et al.,2005). Such conflicting results can be explained by the variability of the endometrial appearance according to the timing of the ultrasound scan (day of human chorionic gonadotropin administration, day of oocyte pick-up or day of embryo transfer). It seems that the most promising data are obtained when the study is performed on the day of human chorionic gonadotropin (hCG) administration, since progesterone production does not interfere with endometrial characteristics at this period of the menstrual cycle.

2.4 Uterine artery blood flow

The introduction of transvaginal Doppler ultrasound makes the measurement of uterine artery blood flow possible, with hope that uterine arterial resistance changes might reflect receptivity of endometrium (Fleischer et al., 1991; Goswamy et al., 1988; Steer et al., 1994;). Color Doppler signals are measured at the uterine arteries and their ascending branches located in the outer third of the myometrium.

Steer et al.(1994) used transvaginal color Doppler to study the uterine arteries in 23 normally cycling women, and they found that the lowest pulsatility index (PI) occurred 9 days after the LH peak. This indicates that the maximum uterine perfusion occurs at about the time of expected implantation. Another index of blood flow, the resistance index, was measured on the day of embryo transfer in a series of women undergoing IVF, and it was found to be lower in those who subsequently became pregnant.

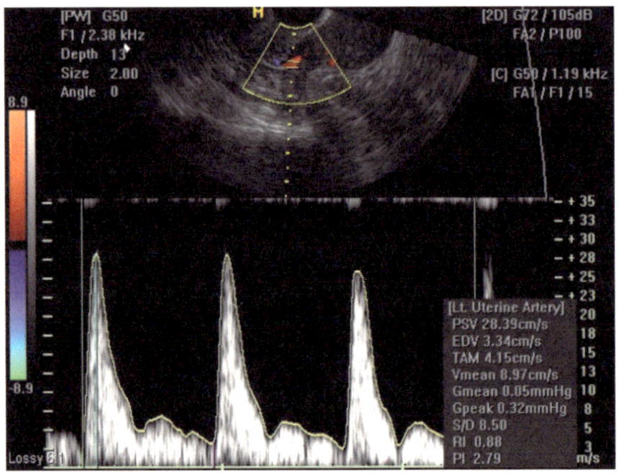

Photo 4. Arteria uterine blood flow

Doppler Studies have demonstrated the uterine and endometrial arteries resistance decreases significantly during the mesoluteal phase, i.e. in the period of embryo implantation (Agrawal et al., 1999; Bourne et al., 1996; Scholtes et al., 1989; Sladkevicius et al., 1993; Tan et al., 1996). It is probable that these vascular changes play a significant role in the implantation process because they are present from the beginning of the embryo nidation.

Sterzik et.al (1989) reported that the resistance index measured on the day of embryo transfer in IVF cycles was significantly lower in patients who subsequently became pregnant as compared with those who failed to achieve pregnancy.

Steer et al. (1992) have used transvaginal color Doppler to study the uterine arterial blood flow in 82 women undergoing IVF on the day of embryo transfer. The PI was calculated and the patients were grouped according to whether the PI was low (1-1.99), medium (2-2.99) or high (3.0+). There were no pregnancies in the high PI group and the PI was significantly lower in the women who become pregnant as compared with those who did not. However, although measurement of uterine artery blood flow impedance on the day of embryo transfer may be able to predict pregnancy, it would be more useful to detect flow abnormalities earlier in the cycle. To investigate this Zaidi et al.(1996) recently measured uterine artery PI in 135 women undergoing IVF on the day of hCG injection. They found significantly lower implantation rates in women with uterine artery PI > 3.0. The authors suggested that the PI on the day of embryo transfer could be used to alter the management, such that a high value (> 3) would lead to elective freezing of the embryos for transfer at a later date in a more favorable cycle. If the PI is normal, the number of embryos transferred could be reduced to minimize the risk of a multiple pregnancy.

The ability of Color Doppler - PI to predict uterine receptivity presents high sensitivity (96-100%) and a high negative predictive value (88-100%) although it has low specificity (13-35%) and positive predictive value (44-56%) (Friedler et al., 1996). Inadequate blood flow would thus prevent implantation, although optimal uterine profusion does not always imply pregnancy. In addition to this, high uterine resistance is observed in less than 10% of non-conception cycles, suggesting that this parameter is responsible for implantation failure in very few cases (Caccitore et al., 1996).

In our study, uterine artery and arcuate artery blood flow were measured with color Doppler ultrasonography at the hCG day. The average values of right or left uterine and intraovarian artery PI, RI, and Vs values were used in the analysis. In the pregnant group average uterine artery PI and RI were significantly lower than in the non-pregnant group. Arcuate artery RI in the pregnant group was significantly lower than that in the non-pregnant group. (Table 3).

In our results, there were statistically significant lower mean uterine artery PI and RI, arcuate artery in the pregnant group than in the non-pregnant group ($P< 0.05$). Arcuate artery PI value was lower in the pregnant group than in the non-pregnant group, but this did not reach statistical significance. Peak systolic velocity (Vs) values in both the mean uterine artery and arcuate artery were higher in the pregnant group than in the non-pregnant group; however, the difference was not statistically significant.

Vascular impedance was calculated with PI, RI, and Vs values, among which PI was found to be the most important. Optimal uterine receptivity can be accomplished by reduced vascular resistance and increased blood flow, which will improve pregnancy success. We suggest the use of transvaginal color Doppler ultrasonography to measure the blood flow in uterine arteries, arcuate arteries before hCG in IVF cycles.

	Doppler values				
Prameter	**(29) BHCG +**	**(56) BHCG -**	**t**	**Z**	**p**
RI Aut HCG	0.71 ± 0.06	0.89 ± 0.07	-6.65		0.000***
PI Aut HCG	1.83 ± 0.14	2.19 ± 0.27		-4.79	0.000***
PVs Aut HCG	21.11 ± 3.47	0.83 ± 0.07	3.04		0.003**
RI a.arcuata HCG	0.56 ± 0.05	0.71 ± 0.06	-3.69		0.000***
PI a.arcuata HCG	1.07 ± 0.09	1.29 ± 0.09	-4.09		0.000***
P Vs a.arcuata	11.07 ± 2.71	7.19 ± 2.94	-3.17		0.004**

**p<0.01 ***p < 0.001

Table 3. Average Doppler values in pregnant and non-pregnant group on HCG day

Although pregnancy outcome tended to be poor in patients with higher mean uterine arterial impedance indices, the predictive value of using a specific resistance index (RI) or pulsatility index (PI) variable in assessing endometrial receptivity seems to be limited (Tekay et al., 1996; Friedler et al., 1996). One of the explanations is that the major uterine compartment is the myometrium and not the endometrium, and thus most of the blood passing through the uterine arteries never reaches the endometrium. These contradictory results are due to significant methodological variations such as the ovarian stimulation protocol used, the cycle's day when the Doppler study was carried out or the sonographic examination route (Merce et al., 2000). A more logical approach would be to evaluate the vascularization around the endometrium directly in an attempt to assess endometrial receptivity.

2.5 Endometrial / subendometrial blood flow

The assessment of the endometrial receptivity is the key for success of all ART procedures. Angiogenesis plays a critical role in various female reproductive processes such as development of a dominant follicle, formation of corpus luteum, endometrial growth and implantation (Demir et al., 2006; Nardo, 2005; Sherer and Abulafia, 2001). For this reason many researches have paid attention to ovarian and uterine/ endometrial vascularization for predicting outcome in IVF programs (Tekay et al., 1995). Invent of the Doppler in ultrasound has significantly improved the understanding of morphological changes occurring in the ovary and the uterus as a reflection of biochemical changes during the menstrual cycle. The vascular changes are reflection of the biochemical changes and can be studied by color Doppler. The spectral/pulse Doppler values give objective assessment of the endometrial vascularity. Therefore, color and pulse Dopplers speak about functional maturity of the endometrium. 3D ultrasound and 3D power Doppler assesses the global vascularity, as compared to vascularity in a single plane on 2D ultrasound and so may give better idea about follicular maturity and endometrial receptivity and therefore implantation rates.

A good blood supply towards the endometrium is usually considered to be an essential requirement for implantation and therefore assessment of endometrial blood flow in IVF treatment has attracted a lot of attention in recent years.

Doppler study allows us to evaluate endometrial blood flow by means of analyzing flow velocity waveforms of subendometrial and endometrial arteries (Achiron et al., 1995; Battaglia et al., 1997; Ivanovski et al., 2007b; Merce et al., 1995; Schild et al., 2001; Yuval et al., 1999; Zaidi et al., 1995) and the color mapping by two-dimensional (Applebaum, 1995; Battaglia et al., 1997;Chien et al., 2002; Yang et al., 1999; Zaidi et al., 1995) or three-dimensional ultrasound (Jarvela et al., 2005; Kupesic et al., 2001; Ng et al., 2006; Wu et al., 2003).

Blood vessels of the uterus and endometrium can be detected by color and power Doppler ultrasound where endometrium and myometrium constitute an anatomical and functional unit. Uterine arteries branch off the internal iliac arteries. Ultrasonically, they look like hyperechoic structures running along the cervix and the isthmic part of the uterus. Arcuate arteries are tortuotic anechoic structures that spread through myometrium. Radial arteries penetrate vertically the myometrial layers of smooth muscle cells and divides after passing through the myometrial-endometrial junction to form the basal arteries that supply the basal portion of the endometrium, and the spiral arterioles that continue up toward the endometrial surface and supply stratum functionale of endometrium. Their shape and size change during menstrual cycle and they shed during menstruation together with the glandular tissue. During pregnancy, these arteries become uteroplacental decidual arteries. Basal arterioles supply endometrial stratum basale. The vessels in genital tract undergo cyclic changes dictated by the hormonal cycle.

At the myometrial- endometrial junction, a specific subendometrial area can be identified as a thin hypoechoic layer between the echogenic endometrium and myometrium on ultrasound examination (McCarthy et al., 1989; Scoutt et al., 1991; Tetlow et al., 1999). Different authors ascribe different names to this layer: junctional zone, inner myometrium, subendometrial halo and subendometrial layer are all synonymous. The layer can be viewed by either ultrasound or MR (Killick, 2007). Histological studies have confirmed that the subendometrial halo surrounding the endometrium represents the innermost layer of the myometrium, and compared with the outer myometrium, it consists of a distinct compartment of more tightly packed muscle cells with increased vascularity (Lesny et al., 1999; Turnbull et al., 1995), suggesting a modified function. Many studies have shown that interactions between the junctional zone and the endometrium may play an important role in the implantation process (Chien et al., 2002; Salle et al., 1998).

Conventionally, pulsed and color Doppler have been used to assess uterine and endometrial blood flow. However, conflicting results have been reported.

Subendometrial radial arteries pulsatility was the only parameter that improved in those cycles where pregnancy was achieved after a previous non-conceptional cycle, except when implantation failed and subsequently a miscarriage or ectopic pregnancy was diagnosed (Merce et al., 1995; Merce et al., 2000a, 2000b).

While some authors (Kupesic et al., 2001) have found that vascular resistance in the endometrial spiral arteries or the subendometrial radial arteries, also called intramyometrial subendometrial arteries (Merce et al., 1995; Merce et al., 2000) was significantly lower on the day of oocyte retrieval or embryo transfer in patients who achieve pregnancy (Battaglia et al., 1997;Ivanovski et al., 2004; Kupesic et al., 2001) others have found no differences (Schild et al., 2001; Yuval et al., 1999; Zaidi et al., 1995).

Now, with the advance of ultrasonography, color Doppler energy imaging has been used in endometrial blood flow assessment. Color Doppler energy is a technology based on the total integral of energy frequency spectrum. It visualizes blood flow with the energy of moving reflectors and enjoys the advantages of high sensitivity to slow blood flow, while being less dependent on angles and providing a less cluttered image. In general, endometrial color mapping has been evaluated in a subjective way although the color area can also be quantified (Yang et al., 1999).

Color mapping of endometrial vascularity can be classified in various types according to the degree of penetration into the endometrial thickness, using conventional color (Applebaum, 1995; Battaglia et al., 1997; Zaidi et al., 1995) or power Doppler (Merce et al., 2002).

The zones of vascularity are defined according to Applebaum (1995) as: zone 1 when the vascularity on power Doppler is seen only in the myometrium surrounding the endometrium; zone 2 when vessels penetrate through the hyperechogenic endometrial edge; zone 3 when it reaches internal hypoechogenic zone and zone 4 when they reach the endometrial cavity.

The absence of color mapping of the endometrium and subendometrial areas means an absolute implantation failure (Zaidi et al., 1995) or a significant decrease (80) of the implantation rate. Conversly, the pregnancy rate increases when the vessels reach the subendometrial halo and endometrium (Zaidi et al., 1995; Chien et al., 2002). The presence of vessels within the endometrium is associated with a thicker endometrium, which suggests a correlation between the endometrial perfusion and endometrial growth. On the other hand, the absence of endometrial-subendometrial blood flow is accompanied by a high uterine artery resistance (Chien et al., 2002).

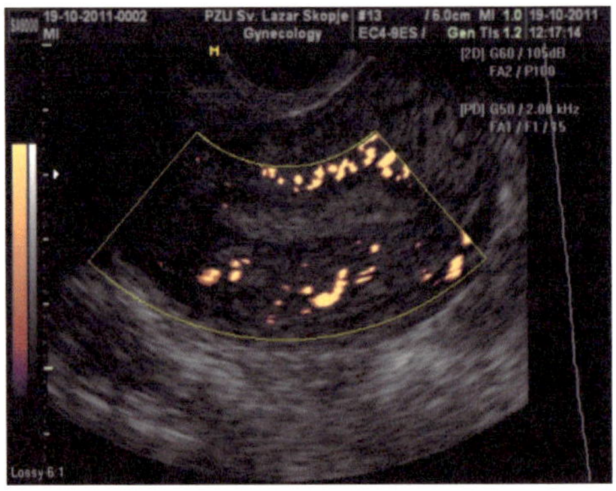

Photo 5. Zone 1 of vascularity

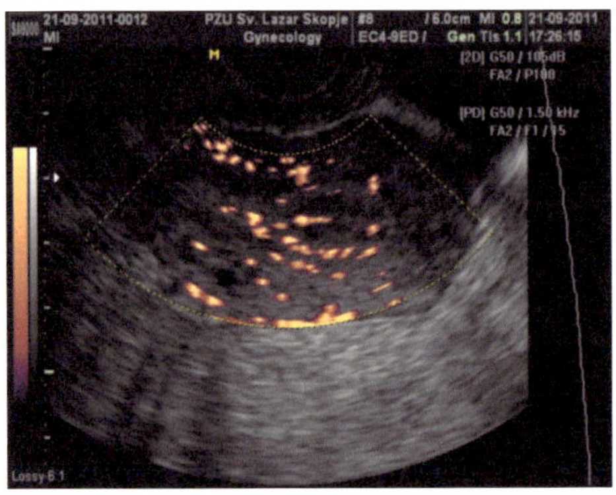

Photo 6. Zone 4 of vascularity

We investigated the correlation of blood flow in the endometrial- subendometrial region detected by Power Doppler sonography with pregnancy outcome of an IVF-ET program. The endometrial-subendometrial blood flow distribution pattern was determined by demonstrating pulsatile color signals in the subendometrial and endometrial regions. For those with vascularization penetrating the subendometrial area, we adopted the definition from Applebaum (1999), summarized as follows: group1, vessels penetrating the outer hypoechogenic area surrounding the endometrium but not entering the hyperechogenic outer margin; group 2, vessels penetrating the hyperechogenic outer margin of the endometrium but not entering the hypoechogenic inner area; and group 3: vessels entering the hypoechogenic inner area in endometrial cavity.

The degree of vascular penetration into the endometrium in relation to pregnancy outcome is shown in Table 4. Although pregnancy rates were significantly higher in patients with group 3 penetration compared with group 1 (P<0.001) or group 2 penetration, there was no significant difference between the groups with zone 1 and zone 2 penetration. There were also significant differences in miscarriage rate: on group of patients without flow was significantly higher than that of those in group 2 or group 3 (50% vs. 12.5% or 7.14%; P<0.001, respectively).

There was significant correlation between group with higher miscarriage rate (S-; E-) and higher uterine artery PI (> 2,9) and RI (>0.96) values.

	Subend. Flow	Subend. Flow	Vascular penetration		
	Present	Absent	Group 1	Group 2	Group 3
	85	21	23	38	24
BHCG +	36 (42.35%)	4 (19%)	6 (26%)	16 (42%)	14 (53%)
BHCG -	49	17	17	22	10
Miscariage rate			3/6(50%)	2/16(12.5%)	1/14(7.14%)

Table 4. Pregnancy and implantation rates in relation to the presence or absence of subendometrial blood flow and zone of vascular penetration.

The report from Li-Wei Chien et al.(2002) showed that the absence of subendometrial blood flow is associated with poor pregnancy outcome; however, this condition is not indicative of a non-receptive endometrium as suggested in our and other study (Zaidi et al., 1995). Although women with no detectable endometrial/subendometrial flow on the day of ET tend to be older, it is noteworthy that more than half (9 of 14, 54.5%) of pregnancies in such women aborted spontaneously. Although these data suggest that development of the endometrial vessel system may play a role in maintaining pregnancy in the early stages, but the case number is too small to draw any conclusion.

The three-dimensional ultrasound allows studying not only the endometrial volume but also the quantitative assessment of vessels density and blood flow within the endometrium and subendometrial region. Vascularization of tissues within the region of interest can be assessed using 3D Power-Doppler angiography and the VOCAL program (Pairleinter et al., 1999). Using this method, three vascular indexes can be calculated: the Vascularization Index (VI), expressed as percentage, measures the number of color voxels in the studied volume, representing the blood vessels within the tissue. The Flow Index (FI) is the color value of all color voxels, representing average color intensity. And the Vascular-Flow Index (VFI) is the average color value of all grey and color voxels, which represents both blood flow and vascularization. Using the "shell" function it is possible to calculate a volume at different thickness around the predetermined endometrium and estimate the vascularization in this "shell". This allows the assessment of the so called "subendometrial region" 3D US has a very low inter-observer and intra observer variability for calculating endometrial volume, with intraclass correlation coefficients ≥0.97 (Bordes et al., 2002; Key-Mensah et al., 1996; Raine-Fenning et al., 2002b; Yaman et al., 1999). However, this depends on the technique used, being the VOCAL method the most reproducible (Reine-Fenning et al., 2003). This technique has been also found to be highly reproducible for estimating ovarian and endometrial vascularization using 3D PD with intraclass correlation coefficients ≥0.99 for all indexes (Alcazar et al., 2005; Raine-Fenning et al., 2002a; Jarvela et al., 2003).

Endometrial and subendometrial blood flows assessed in the same patients by 3D power Doppler indices are significantly lower in stimulated than in natural cycles. (Ng et al., 2004b) It has also been reported that endometrial and subendometrial blood flow are negatively affected by serum estradiol concentrations, but they are not affected by other factors such as women age, smoking habits, or types of infertility or parity during IVF treatment. (Ng et al., 2006)) This fact could explain that ovarian hyperresponders tend to have lower endometrial and subendometrial blood flows during the early luteal phase (+ 2 hCG day). (Ng et al., 2004a)

A reduced endometrial blood flow after ovulation could be related to an increased uterine contractility (Hauksson et al., 1998) and may lead to endometrial hypoxia during the implantation period (Fischer et al., 1993).

Some authors have provide that subendometrial vascularity indices may behave as predicting factors for pregnancy (Kupesic et al., 2001; Wu et al., 2003), on the other hand other authors prefer to calculate only the 3D power Doppler indices of the endometrium (Merce, Donald School Textbook, 2008). Even though most authors assess both endometrial and subendometrial vascularization as a pregnancy predictor (JARVELA ET AL., 2005; Kupesic et al., 2001; Ng et al., 2006; Wu et al., 2003).

Schild at all.(2000) evaluated 96 patients undergoing IVF program by 3D-PDA. Only subendometrial vascularization was assessed. They found that all 3D-PDA indices were significantly lower in conception with non-conception cycles. However, a great overlapping existed. These findings were the same in a subgroup of patients in which at least two good quality embryos were transferred. Logistic regression revealed that subendometrial FI was the strongest predicting factor of IVF success. No association between uterine artery PI and PSV and IVF outcome was found.

On the other hand, Raine-Fenning (2004) found that endometrial and subendometrial vascularity were significantly reduced in women with unexplained subfertility during the mid-late follicular phase, irrespective of estradiol or progesterone concentrations.

A scoring system reported by Kupesic et al. (2004) for uterine receptivity, done on the day of embryo transfer, shows that subendometrial FI<11 was a cut off limit. No pregnancies occurred when it was <11 and the conception group showed its values of 13.2±2.2. No significant differences were found in subendometrial VI and VPI between conception and non-conception cycles. These results were opposite to those reported by Schild et al. (2000).

Wu at al. (2003) reported that subendometrial VFI was significantly higher in those patients who become pregnant. The best prediction rate was achieved by a subendometrial VFI > 0.24, with a sensitivity of 83.3%, specificity of 88.9%, positive predictive value of 93.8% and negative predictive value of 93.8% and negative predictive value of 72.7%.

Järvelä at al.(2005) evaluated endometrial and subendometrial vascularization by 3D PDA using the VOCAL program with a 15°-rotation step. They did not find differences on endometrial and subendometrial vascularization between conception and non-conception cycles. However, they found than in both conception and non-conception cycles endometrial and subendometrial VI decreased significantly between the two examinations this finding would be in agreement with the findings of Raine-Fenning et al. (2004) in natural cycles, who reported a decrease of endometrial vascularity during the periovulatory period.

Whereas Ng et al (2004) documented a lower endometrial VI and VFI in pregnant group on the day of oocyte retrieval and also a non-significant trend of higher implantation and pregnancy rates in patients with absent subendometrial and endometrial flow. This probably can be explained on the basis that hCG administration/LH peak causes increased uterine artery resistance and hence a decrease in endometrial perfusion on the day of oocyte retrieval. This also correlates with the observation by Ng et al, (2006) which says that subendometrial vascularization flow indices are significantly lower in patients with uterine artery RI≥0,95. Multiple logistic regression analysis showed that from multiple parameters only the number of embryos replaced and endometrial VI significantly improved the chance of pregnancy, but this latter had only a marginal predictive value (odd ratio: 0.87, 95% CI: 0.76–0.99).

These findings are in agreement with those reported by Schild et al.(2000) ; Ng et al (2006); who did not find differences in endometrial/ subendometrial VI, FI and VFI between pregnant and non-pregnant women when at least two good quality embryos was transferred. However, when first one or no good quality embryos were transferred all three endometrial VI, FI and VFI were significantly higher in those women who became pregnant as compared with those who did not. These data could indicate that endometrial vascularization might be a non-relevant factor when good quality embryos are transferred but could be an important factor when no quality embryos are transferred.

These conflicting results might be explained by the fact of different timing when performing 3D-PDA assessment.

Our study, performed on ET day, showed that when endometrial FI was < 20 , 17% of patients became pregnant; FI=20-40, 35% became pregnant and when FI>40, 45% of patients became pregnant. The higher FI values correlate with pregnancy outcome (Table 5).

Also, higher VFI significantly associated with higher pregnancy rates. When endometrial VFI was > 20 . 55.5% patients became pregnant, and when VFI < 2, no conception was seen (Table 6).

End FI/Pregnancy rates	**<20**	**20- 40**	**>40**
BHCG +	6	21	5
BHCG -	31	48	6
Total	35 (17.1%)	60 (35 %)	11 (45%)

Table 5. Endometrial FI and pregnancy rate

End VFI/Pregnancy rates	**<2**	**2- 10**	**11-20**	**>20**
BHCG +	/	20	7	5
BHCG -	10	46	14	4
Total	10	66 (30.3%)	21(33.3%)	9 (55.5%)

Table 6. Endometrial VFI and pregnancy rate

Summary, regarding the role of endometrial and subendometrial vascularity assessment the results of several studies are clearly controversial (Kupesic et al., 2001; Jarvela et al., 2005; Ng et al., 2005; Ng et al., 2006; Wu et al., 2003. An explanation for these controversial findings might be the different design of reported studies, specially the timing of ultrasound evaluation. A consensus about the timing of this technique to be used within an IVF program is needed to establish more precise values for endometrial VI, FI and VFI, in order to design new further prospective studies.

On the other hand, the concept of evaluating uterine receptivity by a uterine score including the endometrial blood flow was first introduced by Applebaum (1995). With the absence of subendometrial blood flow, even in the presence of other favorable parameters, no conception was achieved. By using a similar approach, Salle et al. (1998) calculated a uterine score in the secretory phase of the menstrual cycle preceding IVF. Vascularization was considered to be positive if more than three vessels penetrating the outer hypo-echogenic area surrounding the endometrium could be seen. None of the individual ultrasonographic or Doppler parameters tested was of sufficient accuracy to predict uterine receptivity, whereas the uterine score seemed to be a useful predictor of implantation.

However, research by Ng et al. (2006) reported no relationship between endometrial thickness, morphology and pregnancy outcome. End in a recent study, endometrium pattern, endometrium thickness, and end-diastolic blood flow was shown to be the most effective combination for evaluation of uterine receptivity (Dechaund et al., 2008)). Kupesic et al. (2001) compared the 2-D and 3-D ultrasonographic scoring systems by combining parameters including endometrial thickness, volume, echogenicity, and subendometrial blood flow and found the two systems had similar efficiencies in predicting pregnancy outcome of IVF-ET procedures. Ng at al. (2009) discuss the relationship of endometrial blood flow between those who with a thin (≤8mm) endometrium and those with a low volume (≤ 2.5 ml) endometrium. It was found that 3D power Doppler flow indices of the endometrial and subendometrial regions were significantly lower in patients with a low volume endometrium compared with those with a normal volume endometrium. Endometrial end subendometrial vascularity measured by 3D power Doppler ultrasound was significantly lower ($p \leq 0.003$) in patients with a low volume endometrium, but not in those with a thin endometrium. Merce et al. (2008) conclude that endometrial volume and 3D power Doppler indexes are statistically significant in predicting the cycle outcome.

In summary, although 2D and 3D Doppler ultrasound seems to be very interesting tool for assessing the endometrial/subendometrial blood flow in assisted reproductive treatments, its current clinical value in predicting pregnancy in IVF should be considered as limited in view of the controversial results published to date. Though still larger studies are needed to established more precise ultrasound values/parameters to understand the endometrial physiological status better and achieve better pregnancy rates with ART procedures.

3. Ultrasound and embryo transfer

The vast majority of transferred embryos fail to implant in spite of improvements in ovulation induction, fertilization and embryo cleavage. On average, up to 90% of apparently healthy zygotes transferred in utero are destined to vanish, giving no signs of trophoblastic attachment and production of human chorionic gonadotrophin (HCG) (Nikas et al.,1999) The main variables that affect nidation are related to uterine/endometrial receptivity, embryo quality and the efficiency of embryo transfer.

The Embryo transfer (ET) procedure is the final important step in IVF process. It is a critically important procedure. No matter how good the IVF laboratory culture environment is, the physician can ruin everything with a carelessly performed embryo transfer. The entire IVF cycle depends on delicate placement of the embryos at the proper location of the endometrial cavity with minimal trauma and manipulation.

Apart from embryo quality and the age of the patient, success rates after embryo transfer seem to be mostly dependent on factors that relate to the degree of trauma that is inflicted upon the endometrium and myometrium during the transfer procedure. Rigid catheters, blood contamination of the tip, increased myometrial contraction waves and the level of difficulty in introducing the catheter inside the uterine cavity all tend to reduce the probability of implantation of the embryo (Buckett, 2003;Gonen et al., 1991; Goudas et al., 1998; Fanchin et al., 1998; Levi Setti et al., 2003; Lesny et al., 1998; Mansour et al., 1990; Mansour and Aboulghar, 2002; Meriano et al., 2000; Mirkin et al., 2003; Sallam and Sadek, 2003; Schoolcraft et al., 2001; Visser et al., 1993; Wisanto et al., 1989). Also, pregnancy rates may vary greatly among individual providers (Hearns-Stokes et al., 2000; Karande et al., 1999).

The technique used in the transfer procedure may be of importance by allowing for more or less traumatic procedures. The 'clinical touch' method was first described by Steptoe and Edwards and is a well-known technique for embryo transfer (Steptoe and Edwards, 1976). This technique consists of the insertion of a catheter into the cavity until touching the fundal endometrium, followed by a 5/10 mm retreat and subsequent deposition of the embryos. The difficulties and uncertainties of this method have been widely questioned. One of these uncertainties is related to the fact that transfers based only on the sensitivity of the operator are associated with discrepancies between the presumed and true position of the catheter, especially considering the different levels of clinical experience (Buckett, 2003; Hurley et al., 1991; Levi Setti et al., 2003; Sallam and Sadek, 2003; Woolcott and Stanger, 1997).

Waterstone et al. (1991) suggested that the site of deposition of the embryos within the uterine cavity could have profound effects on success rates. Later this finding was also substantiated by Naaktgeboren (1998). By applying a technique in which the embryos are expelled at a fixed distance from the external os, a remarkable decrease was observed in the variability in success rates among physicians: most physicians approximated the success rates of the best-performing physician (Naaktgeboren et al., 1997, 1998). The wide variability between clinicians working in the same center (which to an extent nullifies the potential difference in the laboratory circumstances) clearly demonstrates the role of the clinician in embryo transfer and the magnitude of problem. A possible explanation for this effect may be that replacing embryos in the middle part of the uterus without touching the fundal endometrium allows for a less traumatic embryo transfer, especially for those physicians who have difficulties with approaching the fundal endometrium gently.

Ultrasound-guided embryo transfer (UGET) during an IVF cycle was initially reported during the mid-1980s (Leong et al., 1986; Strickler et al., 1985) and has gradually become an integral part of the embryo transfer technique for many IVF clinics. The potential advantages of this technique compared with standard embryo transfer (performed by clinical feel) include the ability to visualize the uterocervical angle which may aid with difficult transfers, reliably determine the catheter distance from the fundus at the time of embryo transfer, and visualize any unforeseen uterine abnormalities before the transfer. Some studies have demonstrated a benefit in favor of UGET when compared to embryo transfer without ultrasound guidance (Coroleu et al., 2000; Ivanovski et al., 2006; Matorras et al., 2002; Prapas et al., 2001; Sallam et al., 2002; Tang et al., 2001) although others have not (Al-Shawaf et al., 1993; Garcia-Velasco et al., 2002; Kan et al., 1999). Careful examination of the data from four properly randomized clinical trials (Coroleu et al., 2000; Garcia-Velasco et al., 2002; Matorras et al., 2002; Tang et al., 2001) showed a significant advantage to UGET with regard to implantation, clinical pregnancy, and ongoing pregnancy rates (Buckett, 2003; Sallam and Sadek, 2003).

It has been described that Mock Embryo Transfer (MET) in a cycle preceding the actual IVF procedure or immediately before the actual transfer procedure might provide information about what to expect during the ET and thereby facilitate the procedure (Sharif et al., 1995). In one randomized controlled trial employing the "dummy transfer" it was stated that this procedure could influence the choice of catheter and could improve pregnancy rates (Mansour et al., 1990).

Shamonki at al. (2005a) proposed that ultrasound guided trial transfer (UTT) in the office can be performed as an alternative to UGET for most patients. UTT can theoretically identify those patients with a discrepancy between perceived and actual uterine cavity length in an office setting where logistical issues are of less concern, and thus save UGET for only a select minority of patients where the trial transfer was challenging. The data from their study demonstrate that UTT can be useful method in identifying patients who will otherwise have an inaccurate trial transfer if the procedure were done blindly (Matorras et al., 2002; Sallam et al., 2002). Two studies demonstrated that cavity depth as noted by ultrasound at the time of embryo transfer differed from the cavity depth via office trial transfer by ≥1.0 cm in ≥30% of cases (Pope et al., 2004; Shamonki et al., 2005b). The main risk factor predicting a discrepancy between the perceived and actual uterine cavity length was a history of pregnancy, especially if the patient had a delivery (Shamonki et al., 2005b). Another far less likely theory explaining the discrepancy is that uterine length may be increased with exposure to estradiol. Research has demonstrated a positive correlation between estradiol exposure and uterine size (Adams et al, 1984; Gull et al., 2005). However, if ~2 weeks of high estradiol exposure significantly lengthened the uterus during an IVF cycle, one would expect a more uniform discrepancy between trial transfer and actual uterine cavity lengths in the majority of IVF patients, which is not the case. Physicians may argue that UGET has additional benefits over UTT other than the diagnosis of a trial transfer inaccuracy. The evidence from studies would imply that the addition of ultrasound guidance during trial transfer would further reduce the benefit of UGET when used routinely (Diedrich et al., 1989; Englert et al., 1986; Ghazzawi et al., 1999; Goudas et al., 1998; Hearns-Stokes et al., 2000; Leeton et al., 1982; Wood et al., 1985).

Among the various aspects of embryo transfer, the site of embryo placement in the uterine cavity has been postulated to influence embryo implantation rates. Whereas some investigators believe that higher levels in the endometrial cavity closer to the uterine fundus lead to higher rates (Krampl et al., 1995; Meldrum et al., 1987), others have suggested that improved embryo transfer results are obtained when the embryos are placed at lower levels in the uterine cavity (Coroleu et al., 2002a; Frankfurteret al., 2003; Lesny et al., 1998; Naaktgeboren et al., 1997; Naaktgeboren et al., 1998; Van de Pas et al., 2003; Waterstone et al., 1991; Woolcott and Stanger, 1997;). Waterstone et al. (1991) reported the results of embryo transfer performed by two clinicians who followed different techniques. The first introduced the catheter until he felt the fundus and then pulled it back 5 mm before injecting the embryos, and achieved a final pregnancy rate of 24%. The second clinician introduced the catheter until a depth of 5 cm from the external orifice of the cervix and deposited the embryos without touching the fundus, and obtained a pregnancy rate of 46%. When the first clinician modified his technique according to that of the second, improvement in pregnancy rates was observed. Coroleu et al. (2002) demonstrated in a prospective randomized trial of women undergoing UGET that the pregnancy rate was significantly higher when the embryos were transferred at 1.5–2.0cm instead of at 1.0 cm from the uterine fundus. Frankfurter et al. (2003) retrospectively analyzed 23 patients who underwent two cycles of ultrasound-guided embryo transfer each, considering for each patient a transfer that resulted in pregnancy and one that did not. The results showed better pregnancy rates when the site of embryo placement relative to the length of the endometrial cavity was more distant from the uterine fundus. No significant difference was observed when comparing the absolute distance.

In our study 106 patients underwent a standard down regulation protocol for ovarian stimulation in IVf cycles. Embryo transfer took place 2-4 days after oocyte retrieval. The patients were grouped according to the distance between the tip of the catheter and the uterine fundus at transfer: group 1 : 10 ± 2.5mm; group 2: 15 ± 2.5mm Patients were selected on the basis of the following inclusion criteria; main causes of infertility was tubal, ovaria, idiopatic or male factor and normal uterine cavity confirmed by ultrasound or hysterosalpingography. There were no differences in age, number of days of ovarian stimulation, total number of oocyte retrieved, and number of good quality embryos between these groups of patients. There was statistically significantly difference in pregnancy rate (group 1= 28,8 and group 2= 46,2%) respectively, with ($P<0.05$). Our results suggest that depth of embryo replacement inside the uterine cavity may influence the implantation rates and should be considered as an important factor to improve the success of IVF cycles.

One study retrospectively demonstrated that for every additional millimeter embryos are deposited away from the fundus, as noted by abdominal ultrasound, the odds of clinical pregnancy increased by 11% (Pope et al., 2004). However, not all studies show an association between embryo transfer location and outcome (Rosenlund et al., 1996). In addition, others demonstrate that the best site for embryo transfer is the center of the uterine cavity, and that the relative site of embryo deposition is more important than the actual distance from the fundus (Franco et al., 2004; Oliveira et al., 2004). Finally, some authors postulate that the question regarding the site of embryo transfer does is of no importance since it does not influence implantation as long as embryos are placed in the upper half of the cavity (Nazari et al., 1993; Roselund et al., 1996).

Various studies have suggested implantation in locations ranging from the lower uterine segment, to various distances (0.5cm-2.0cm) from the uterine fundus. However, these distances still only represent generalized locations. Furthermore, the value to place on these distances as guidelines decreases when considering that the configuration and dimensions of the uterine cavity vary between women. The location of embryo transfer in respect to the uterine anatomy also varies among physicians.

Two dimensional sonography has still only provided guidance as to the general area at which the embryo should be released for implantation. 3D sonography can improve visualization of the uterus in patients with normal anatomy and especially in those with congenital uterine anomalies. Thus, the present invention provides a maximal implantation potential (MIP) point as a target for embryo transfers.

The uterine cavity resembles an inverted triangle and the fallopian tubes open into the cavity, one in each of the upper regions of the triangle. The MIP is the intersection of these two imaginary lines, one originating in each fallopian tube, within the inverted triangle. In natural pregnancies, fertilization usually occurs in the ampullary segment of the fallopian tube and the pre-embryo then travels down to the uterus and usually implants in the anterior or posterior segment of the uterus close to its trajectory line, where the endometrium is the thickest and has the greatest blood flow. In patients undergoing IVF, the fallopian tubes are bypassed, placing the embryos directly into the uterus (Gergely et al., 2005).

Liedholm et al. (1980) placed small spheres in a column containing 50 µl of fluid and performed a simulated embryo transfer immediately before hysterectomy. The uterine cavity was then inspected and the microspheres were found within a distance of 1 cm from the presumed deposition site. These results emphasize the importance of the site where the embryos were transferred. Baba et al. (2000) analyzed 60 embryo transfers that resulted in 22 pregnancies and 32 gestational sacs. Twenty-six of the 32 sacs were detected by three-dimensional ultrasound in the area where the air bubble had been observed immediately after transfer.

From early work on surgically removed uteri of Adams et al. (1956) implantation was found to take place in the upper half of the uterine cavity, most on the posterior wall of the uterus. This further supports the MIP point as an advantageous spot, mimicking implantation in the general population. Since 3D/4D ultrasonography allows us to identify the MIP point with great ease, it is now possible to use the combination of MIP and 3D/4D sonography to accomplish embryo transfers accurately. Thus, the Maximal Implantation Potential Point can be readily identified and individualized for each patient. By using the MIP point, placement of the embryos occurs where nature intended. Because of individual anatomic differences, the MIP point can be individually tailored. Further advances in 3D ultrasonography as well as the introduction of 4D sonography have enabled us to visualize the transfer catheter in real time as it moves towards its target, the MIP point. Embryo transfers at the MIP were associated with good implantation and pregnancy rates (Gergely et al., 2005).

It is not fully understood why the pregnancy rate is higher with the transfer of embryos lower in the uterine cavity. One theory suggests that catheter contact with the uterine fundus may be avoided when embryos are transferred to the lower part of the uterine cavity. Strong fundo-uterine contractions can result from fundal contact (Fanchin et al., 1998; Lesny et al., 1998), which may have a negative impact on pregnancy rates (Lesny et al., 1999). It is inevitable that insertion of the catheter- after all a foreign body- may interfere with normal uterine peristalsis. Embryos often relocate from the uterine cavity after IVF/ET. They have been found in the vagina (Poindexter et al., 1986; Schulman et al., 1986) and there is a high ectopic pregnancy rate, raging from 2.1% (Azem et al., 1993) to 9.4% (Zouves et al., 1991) after assisted conception treatment. It is worth remembering that the very first pregnancy conceived after IVF/ET was an ectopic gestation in the fallopian tube (Steptoe and Edwards, 1976). The evidence that this relocation is the consequence of junctional zone contractions is considerable. Experimental studies of mock ET in humans have demonstrated the expulsion of methylene blue in 57% of transfers (Mansouret al., 1994) and the movement of X-ray contrast medium towards the fallopian tubes and cervix/vagina in 38% and 21%, respectively (Knutzen et al., 1992). In observations of junctional zone contractions after easy and difficult mock ETs,(Lesny et al., 1998) use of different catheters,(63) application of a tenaculum to the cervix (lesny et al., 1999a) or stimulation of contractions after transmyometrial ET (Biervliet et al., 2002; Lesny et al., 1999b) all report increased contractions following increasing trauma at the time of ET. Using mock ET in oocyte donor patients as a model, it was shown that even minimal stimulation such as touching the uterine fundus with the soft end of the ET catheter is capable of generating evident contractions, which can relocate mock embryos (a bolus of the echogenic substance Echovist) from the upper part of the uterine cavity towards the cervix or into the fallopian tubes.

There are only limited data from studies concerning the speed of withdrawal of the catheter. Some authors have suggested that it is preferable to wait before retiring the catheter so that the uterus can become stabilized (Wisanto et al., 1989), whereas others report good results withdrawing the catheter immediately after an easy transfer (Zech et al., 1997). No differences were observed in the pregnancy rate between withdrawals of the catheter immediately after embryo deposit or after a 30 s wait in a population of women with good response to stimulation and "easy" US- guided embryo transfer on at least two optimal embryos (Martinez et al., 2001).

Various catheter types exist. They can be rigid or soft, with or without outer catheter, with or without metal sound catheter, with or without "memory". Coroleu et al. (2006) In a pilot study suggested that the use of the echogenic Wallace catheter simplifies ultrasound-guided embryo transfer as it facilitates catheter identification under ultrasound, and thus the duration of the embryo transfer procedure was significantly shorter in the echogenic catheter group as compared with the standard catheter group. However, they could not find a definite benefit in terms of pregnancy rates. In contrast, the use of the new catheter was associated with a significant increase in the number of twin pregnancies.

Several randomized and non-randomized studies have been performed to compare different brands of catheters (Mansour et al., 1990; Gonen et al., 1991; Wisanto et al., 1989). Soft catheters seem to lead to superior results, but insertion can be more difficult. Furthermore, the use of a soft catheter instead of a rigid one may cause less endometrial trauma and has been shown to improve outcome (Wood et al., 2000).

Four of the randomized controlled trials (Garcia-Velasco et al., 2002; Matorras et al., 2002; Sallam et al., 2002; Tang et al., 2001;) reported more ectopic pregnancies in the blind group than in the ultrasound-assisted ET group. Three randomized controlled trials did not mention ectopic pregnancies. One study retrospectively demonstrated that ectopic pregnancies occurred significantly less frequently when the embryos were placed away from the fundus (Pope et al., 2004).

The main disadvantages of using ultrasound guidance during embryo transfer is patient discomfort due to a full bladder. Some authors claim that a full bladder, required for UGET, can make the embryo transfer easier because this reduces the angle at the cervico-uterine junction and straightens the uterine cavity in relation to the cervical canal (Sharif et al., 1995; Sundstrom et al., 1984; Wood et al., 2000). When comparing a full bladder without the use of ultrasound during embryo transfer, some data have shown a benefit (Lewin et al., 1997) while others have not (Mitchell et al., 1989). In their study Lorusso et al., (2005); Kosmas et al. (2007) shows that high overall pregnancy rates can be achieved when ETs are performed in patients with an empty bladder, whether they are performed under ultrasound guidance or not. Also, studies that utilize transvaginal ultrasound, requiring an empty bladder during embryo transfer, show an improvement in the pregnancy rate (Anderson et al., 2002; Kojima et al., 2001; Lindheim et al., 1999) suggesting that a full bladder required for UGET is not a confounder for improving outcome.

The majority of the published studies were done with abdominal ultrasound.. The value of abdominal ultrasound in addition of visualizing the catheter is to straighten the uterovesical angle which my make the insertion of the catheter easier (Sallam et al., 2000). Kojima et al. (2001) tried to use vaginal ultrasound as it allows visualization of the tip of the catheter precisely and concluded that it increases the pregnancy and implantation rate; in the same time they admitted that it technically more difficult. The procedure did not gain popularity because of its discomfort to the patient. Isobe et al. (2003) compared the transrectal approach in retroflexed uterus and found that it increases the incidence of easier transfer and pregnancy rate; however, there was no comment on the acceptance of the procedure.

We believe that gentle and atraumatic ET is the simplest and cheapest way to improve disappointing pregnancy rates. In our routine clinical practice ET is performed by : transabdominal ultrasound guided with full bladder; with soft catheters; not touching the uterine fundus - distance between the tip of the catheter and the uterine fundus > 1.5 cm ; not using a tenaculum; utilizing a mock ET…

3.1 Conclusion

Of all factors influencing the ET process, ultrasound guidance of the ET has been studied the most over the past decade. Issues related to the ET technique, ET provider/physician, transferred embryos and unloading site in the uterus and their relationship to ultrasound guidance were the most debatable aspects of the process.

In summary, the reports regarding the effect of guiding the transferred embryo deposition by ultrasound are conflicting. Some showing an improvement in outcome (Al-Shawaf et al., 1993; Baba et al., 2000; Ivanovski et al., 2006; Kan et al., 1999; Kojima et al., 2001;Woolcott et al., 1998), others demonstrating no difference (Coroleu et al., 2002; De Camargo et al., 2004; Garcia-Velasco et al., 2002; Li et al., 2005; Lindheim et al., 1999; Mirkin et al., 2003; Prapas et al., 1995) and others with mixed results (Fisser et al., 2006; Hurley et al., 1991; Prapas et al., 2001). No study has shown a worsening of outcome when ultrasonography is used.

Compared with the traditional method, abdominal ultrasound-guided embryo transfer has a number of potential benefits (Hearns-Stokes et al., 2000; Leeton et al., 1982; Nabi et al., 1997; Sallam et al., 2002). First, with the guidance of ultrasound, the catheter can be bent to easily pass through the cervical canal and follow the uterine axis, which helps avoid overstimulation and reduction in incidence of difficult transfers, endometrial trauma (Letterie et al., 1999; Woolcott and Stanger, 1997), and bleeding (Goudas et al., 1998; Nabi et al., 1997; Sallam et al., 2002) that can cause excessive fundo-uterine contractions (Lesny et al., 1999) at the time of embryo transfer has been associated with lower clinical pregnancy rates (Goudas et al., 1998; Sallam et al., 2002). Second, the entire process of catheterization and release of the embryos can be visualized, making it easier to place the embryos in the correct position within the uterus (Woolcott and Stanger, 1997) and decrease the chance of improper embryo placement (Coroleu et al., 2002; Pope et al., 2004; Rosenlund et al., 1996; Shamonki et al., 2005; Woolcott and Stanger, 1997). The 3D US allows viewing the catheter tip in a frontal as well as a sagittal and transverse plans, thus it facilitates precise embryo placement inside the uterus. In addition, the full bladder required for transabdominal ultrasound itself is useful for the correction of uterine access through the cervical route in cases of pronounced anteversion–anteflexion. Because of individual anatomic differences the maximal implantation potential point should be readily identified and individualized for each patient.

In particular, the main disadvantages of using ultrasound guidance during embryo transfer may be the additional time and personnel required, as well as patient discomfort due to a full bladder and the urge to urinate (Bucket et al., 2003)

4. References

Achiron R, Levran D, Sivan E, Lipitz S, Dor J, Mashiach S. (1995) Endometrial blood flow response to hormone replacement therapy in women with premature ovarian failure: a transvaginal Doppler study. Fertile steril; 63;550-4

Adams EC, Hertig AT, Rock J. (1956) A description of 34 human ova within the first 17 days of development. Am J Anat; 98:435–93.

Adams J, Mason WP, Tucker M, Morris DV and Jacobs HS (1984) Ultrasound assessment of changes in the ovary and the uterus during LHRH therapy. Upsala J Med Sci89,39–42.

Agrawal R, Conway GS, Sladikevicius p, payne NN, Bekir J, Campbell S et al. (1999) Serum vascular endothelial growth factor (VEGF) in the normal menstrual cycle: association with changes in ovarian and uterine Doppler blood flow. Clin Endocrinol 9Oxf); 50:101-6

Alcázar, JL. (2006) Three-dimensional ultrasound assessment of endometrial receptivity: a review. Reproductive Biology and Endocrinology; 4:56-59

Alcázar JL, Mercé LT, García-Manero M, Bau S, López-García G: (2005) Endometrial volume and vascularity measurements by transvaginal three-dimensional ultrasonography and power Doppler angiography in stimulated and tumoral endometria: an inter-observer reproducibility study. J Ultrasound Med, 24:1091-1098.

Al-Shawaf T, Yang D, al-Magid Y, Seaton A, Iketubosin F, Craft I (1993). Ultrasonic monitoring during replacement of frozen/thawed embryos in natural and hormone replacement cycles. Hum Reprod;8:2068-74.

Amir W, Micha B, Ariel H, Liat LG, Jehoshua D, Adrian S. (2007) Predicting factors for endometrial thickness during treatment with assisted reproductive technology. Fertil Steril; 4: 799- 804.

Anderson RE, Nugent NL, Gregg AT, Nunn SL and Behr BR (2002) Transvaginal ultrasound-guided embryo transfer improves outcome in patients with previous failed in vitro fertilization cycles. Fertil Steril77,769–775.

Applebaum M. (1995) The Menstrual Cycle, menopause, Ovulation Induction, an In Vitro fertilization. In: Copel JA, reed KL (Eds): Doppler Ultrasound in Obsterics and Gynecology. New York: raven Press,; 71-86

Applebaum M. (1995) The uterine biophysical profile. Ultrasound Obstet Gynecol;5:67–8.

Azem F, Yaron Y, Botchan A (1993). Ectopic pregnancy after in vitro fertilization -embryo transfer (IVF/ET): the possible role of the ET technique. J Assist Reprod Genet;10:302- 304.

Baba K, ishiara O, hayashi N, saitoh M, Taya j, Kinoshita K. (2000) Where does the embryo implant after embryo transfer in humans. Fertil steril; 73:123-5

Baba K, Ishihara O, Hayashi N, Saitoh M, Taya J, Kinoshita K. (2000) Three-dimensional ultrasound in embryo transfer. Ultrasound Obstet Gynecol;16:372–3.

Bakos O, Lundvist O, Bergh T. (1993) Transvaginal sonographic evaluation of endometrial growth and texture in spontaneous ovulatory cycles - a descriptive study. Hum Reprod; 8: 799-806

Bassil S. (2001) Changes in endometrial thickness, width, length and pattern in predicting pregnancy outcome during ovarian stimulation in in vitro fertilization. Ultrasound Obstet Gynecol; 18:258-63

Battaglia C, Artini PG, Giulini S, salvatori M, maxia N, Petraglia F et al. (1997) Color Doppler changes and tromboxane production after ovarian stimulation with gonadotrophin-releasing hormone agonist. Hum Reprod; 11:2477-82.

Biervliet FP, Lesny P, Maguiness SD, Robinson J, Killick SR (2002). Transmyometrial embryo transfer and junctional zone contractions. Hum Reprod;17:347- 350.

Blumenfeld Z, Dirnfeld M, Beck H. (1990). Comparasion of treatment of uterine leiomyomata with three GnRH agonistic analogues - efficacy and side-effects. In Vickery B and Lunenfield B (eds.) GnRH Analogues in cancer and Human Reproduction; Vol.3 : 45 (boston: Kluwer Academic Publishers)

Bordes A, Bory AM, Benchaib M, Rudigoz RC, Salle B: (2002) Reproducibility of transvaginal three-dimensional endometrial volume measurements with virtual organ computer-aided analysis (VOCAL) during ovarian stimulation. Ultrasound Obstet Gynecol, 19:76-80.

Bourne TH, Hagstrom HG, Granberg S, Josefsson B, hahlin M, Hellberg P, et all. (1996) Ultrasound studies of vascular and morphological changes in the human uterus after a positive self-test for the urinary luteinizing hormone surge. Hum Reprod; 11:369-5

Buckett WM (2003) A meta-analysis of ultrasound-guided versus clinical touch embryo transfer. Fertil Steril 80, 1037–1041.

Cacciatore, B., Tiitinen, A. and Yhkorkala, O. (1996). Is it possible to improve uterine blood flow in infertile women? [Abstract]; Ultrasound Obstet. Gynecol, 8(Suppl.l), 204

Caccitore B, Simberg N, Fusaro P, Titinen A. (1996) Transvaginal Doppler study of uterine artery blood flow in in-vitro fertilization - embryo transfer cycles. Fertile Steril; 66: 130-4

Check JH, Dietterich C, Lurie D. (2000) Non-homogenous hyperechogenic pattern 3 days after embryo transfer is associated with lower pregnancy rates. Hum Reprod; 15:1096-74.

Check JH, Gandica R, Dietterich C, Lurie D. (2003) Evaluation of a nonhomogeneous endometrial echo pattern in the midluteal phase as a potential factor associated with unexplained infertility. Fertil steril; 79:590-3

Chien LW, Au HK, Chen PL, Xiao J, CR. (2002) Assessment of uterine receptivity by the endometrial-subendometrial blood flow distribution pattern in women undergoing in vitro fertilization-embryo transfer. Fertil Steril; 78:245-251.

Coroleu B, Barri P, Carreras O, Belil I, Buxaderas R, Veiga A, and BalaschJ. (2006) Effect of using an echogenic catheter for ultrasound-guided embryo transfer in an IVF programme: a prospective, randomized, controlled study Hum Reprod; 21: 1809 - 1815.

Coroleu B, Barri PN, Carreras O, Martinez F, Parriego M, Hereter L, Parera N, Veiga A and Balasch J (2002) The influence of the depth of embryo replacement into the uterine cavity on implantation rates after IVF: a controlled, ultrasound-guided study. Hum Reprod17,341–346.

Coroleu B, Barri PN, Carreras O, Martínez F, Veiga A, Balasch J. (2002) The usefulness of ultrasound guidance in frozen-thawed embryo transfer: a prospective randomized clinical trial. Hum Reprod;17:2885–90.

Coroleu B, Carreras O, Veiga A, Martell A, Martinez F, Belil I, Hereter L and Barri PN (2000) Embryo transfer under ultrasound guidance improves pregnancy rates after in-vitro fertilization. Hum Reprod15,616–620.

De Camargo Martins AMV, Baruffi RLR, Mauri AL, Peteresen C, Oliveira JBA, Contart P, et al. (2004) Ultrasound guidance is not necessary during easy transfers. J Assist Reprod Genet;21:421–5.

De Ziegler D, Fanchin R.(1994) Endometrial receptivity in controlled ovarian hyperstimulation (COH): the hormonal factor. In: Bulletti C, Gurpide E, Flagmini C, (eds): the Human Endometrium. Ann n Y Acad Sci; 734: 209-20.

Dechaund H, bessueille E, Bousquet PJ, Reyftman L, Hamamah S, Hedon B (2008). Optimal timing of ultrasonographic and Doppler evaluation of uterine receptivity to implantation. Reprod Biomed Online; 16:368-375.

Demir R, Kayisli UA, Cayli S, Hupperzt B: (2006) Sequential steps during vasculogenesis and angiogenesis in the very early human placenta. Placenta, 27:535-539.

Dickey, R. P., Olar, T. T., Curole, D. N., Taylor, S. N. and Rye, P. H. (1992). Endometrial pat-tern and thickness associated with pregnancy outcome after assisted reproduction technolo-gies. Hum. Reprod.; 7, 418-21

DiedrichK, Van der Ven H, Al-Hasani S and Krebs D (1989) Establishment of pregnancy related to embryo transfer techniques after in-vitro fertilization. Hum Reprod4,111–114.

Dietterich C, Check JH, Choe JK, Nazari A, Lurie D. (2002) Increased endometrial thickness on the day of human chronic gonadotrophin injection does not adversely affect pregnancy or implantation ratios following in vitro fertilization-embryo transfer. Fertil Steril; 4: 781-6.

Edwards RG. (1995). Clinical approaches to increasing uterine receptivity during human implantation. Hum Reprod;10(Suppl 2):60-6.

EnglertY, Puissant F, Camus M, Van Hoeck J and Leroy F (1986) Clinical study on embryo transfer after human in vitro fertilization. J in Vitro Fertil Embryo Transfer3,243–246.

Fanchin R, Righini C, Ayoubi JM, Olivennes F, de Ziegler D, Frydman R. (2000) New look at endometrial echogenicity: objective computer-assisted measurements predict endometrial receptivity in in vitro fertilization-embryo transfer. Fertil Steril; 2: 274-81.

Fanchin R. (2001) Assessing uterine receptivity in 2001. Ultrasonographic glances at the New Millennium. An N Y Acad Sci; 943;185-202

Fanchin, R., Righini, C., Olivennes, F., Taylor, S., Ziegler de, D. and Frydman, R. (1998) Uterine contractions at the time of embryo transfer alter pregnancy rates after in-vitro fertilization. Hum. Reprod., 13, 1986–1974.

Fischer B, bavister BD. (1993) Oxygen tension in the oviduct and uterus of rhesus monkeys, hamsters and rabbits. J Reprod Fertil; 99:673-9.

Fleischer, A. C, Herbert, C. M., Sacks, G. A, YVentz, A. C, Entman, S. S. and James, A. E. Jr (1986). Sonography of the endometrium during conception and nonconception cycles of in vitro fertilization and embryo transfer. Fertil. Steril; 46, 442-7

Fleischer, A. C, Herbert, C. M., Sacks, G. A., Wentz, A. C. and Entman, S. S. (1986) Non-conception cvcles of IVF-ET. Fertil. Steril; 46, 442-6

Fleischer, A.C., Herbert, C.M., Hill, G.A. et al. (1991) Transvaginal sonography of the endometrium during induced cycles. J. Ultrasound Med; 10, 93–95.

Flisser E, Grifo JA, Krey LC, Noyes N. (2006) Transabdominal ultrasound-assisted embryo transfer and pregnancy outcome. Fertil Steril;85:353–7.

Forrest, T. S., Elvaderani, M. K., Muilenburg, M. I., Bewtra, C, Kable, W. T. and Sullivan, P. (1988) Cyclic endometrial changes: ultrasound assessment with histologic correlation. Radiol-ogy; 167, 233-7

Franco JG Jr, Martins AM, Baruffi RL, Mauri AL, Petersen CG, Felipe V, Contart P,Pontes A, Oliveira JB. (2004) Best site for embryo transfer: the upper or lower half of endometrial cavity? Hum Reprod ;19:1785-1790.

Frankfurter D, Silva CP, Mota F, Trimarchi JB and Keefe D (2003) The transfer point is a novel measure of embryo placement. Fertil Steril 79, 1416–1421

Frankfurter D, Trimachi J, Silva C, Keefe D. (2004) Middle to lower uterine segment embryo transfer improves implantation and pregnancy rates compared with fundal embryo transfer. Fertil Steril; 81:1273–7.

Freidler, S., Schenker, J. G., Herman, A. and Lewin, A. (1996) The role of ultrasonographv in the evaluation of endometrial receptivity fol-lowing assisted reproductive treatments: a crit-ical review. Hum. Reprod. Update; 2, 323-35

Fujiwara T, Togashi K, Yamaoka T, Nakai A, Kido A, Nishio S, yamamoto T, Kitagaki H, Fujii S (2004). Kinematiks of the uterus: Cine mode MR Imaging. Radiographics; 24: 19-26

Garcia-Velasco JA, Isaza V, Martinez-Salazar J, Landazabal A, Requena A, Remohi J and Simon C (2002) Transabdominal ultrasound-guided embryo transfer does not increase pregnancy rates in oocyte recipients. Fertil Steril 78,534–539.

Gergely RZ, DeUgarte CM, Danzer H, Surrey M, Hill D, DeCherney AH.(2005) Three dimensional/four dimensional ultrasoundguided embryo transfer using the maximal implantation potential point. Fertility and Sterility 84: 500-503).

GhazzawiIM, Al-Hasani S, Karaki R and Souso S (1999) Transfer technique and catheter choice influence the incidence of transcervical embryo expulsion and the outcome of IVF. Hum Reprod14,677–682.

Glissant, A., de Mouzon, J. and Frydman, R. (1985) Ultrasound study of the endometrium during in vitro fertilization cycles. Fertil. Steril; 44, 786-90

Goldberg BB, Liu JB, Kuhlman K, Merton DA, Kurtz AB.(1991). Endoluminal gynecologic ultrasound: preliminary results. J Ultrasound Med; 10: 583-90

Gonen, Y., Casper, R. F., Jacobson, W. and Blankier, J. (1989). Endometrial thickness and growth during ovarian stimulation: a possible predictor of implantation in in vitro fertiliza-tion. Fertil. Steril, 52, 446-50

Gonen, Y., Dirnfeld, M., Goldman, S., Koifman, M. and Abramovici, H. (1991) Does the choice of catheter for embryo transfer influence the success rate of in-vitro fertilization? Hum. Reprod., 6, 1092–1094.

Goswamy RK, Williams G, Steptoe PC. (1988) Decreased uterine perfusion—a cause of infertility. Hum Reprod; 3:955–9.

Goudas, V.T., Hammitt, D.G., Damario, M.A., Session, D.R., Singh, A.P. and Dumesic, D.A. (1998) Blood on the embryo transfer catheter is associated with decreased rates of embryo implantation and clinical pregnancy with the use of in vitro fertilization–embryo transfer. Fertil. Steril., 70, 878–882.

Gull B, Karlsson B, Milsom I and Granberg S (2001) Factors associated with endometrial thickness and uterine size in a random sample of postmenopausal women.Am J Obstet Gynecol,185,386–391.

Hauksson A, Akerlund M, Melin P. (1988) Uterine blood flow and myometrial activity at menstruation, and the action of vasopressin and a synthetic antagonist. Br J Obstet Gynecol; 95:898-904.

Hearns-Stokes, R.M., Miller, T.B., Scott, L., Creuss, D., Chakraborty, P.K. and Segars, J.H. (2000) Pregnancy rates after embryo transfer depend on the provider at embryo transfer. Fertil. Steril., 74, 80–86.

Hurley VA, Osborn JC, Leoni MA, Leeton J. (1991) Ultrasound-guided embryo transfer: a controlled trial. Fertil Steril;55:559–62.

Isobe T, Minoura H, Kawato H and Toyoda N. (2003) Validity of trans-rectal ultrasound-guided embryo transfer against retroflexed uterus Reprod Med Biol; 2: 159–163.

Ivanovski M, Lazarevski S, Popovic M et al. (September 2004). Assessment of endometrial receptivity by transvaginal Color Doppler in women undergoing IVF-ET procedures. 1-st Balkan Congress of reproductive Medicine. Thessaloniki, Greece. Book of Abstracts ; p 2.

Ivanovski M, lazarevski S, Popovic M et al.(2007b). Comparison of blood flow measured by Doppler ultrasound between natural and stimulated ovulatory cycles in in vitro fertilization and embryo transfer program. VOX Medici; 57:28-31

Ivanovski M, lazarevski S, Popovik M et al.(2007a). Assessment of endometrial thickness and pattern in prediction of pregnancy in an in vitro fertilization an embryo transfer cycles after ovarian stimulation. Macedonian medical review; 4-6:117-124

Ivanovski M. (November 2006). Comparison of ultrasound guided embryo transfer and previous failed blind embryo transfer in IVF cycles. XVIII FIGO World Congress of Gynecology and Obstetrics; Kuala Lumpur, Malaysia; Book of abstracts: 160.

Jarvela IY, Sladkevicius P, Kelly S, Ojha K, Campbell S, Nargund G: (2005) Evaluation of endometrial receptivity during in-vitro fertilization using three-dimensional power Doppler ultrasound. Ultrasound Obstet Gynecol, 26:765-769.

Jarvela IY, Sladkevicius P, Tekay AH, Campbell S, Nargund G: (2003) Intraobserver and interobserver variability of ovarian volume, gray-scale and color flow indices obtained using transvaginal three-dimensional power Doppler ultrasonography. Ultrasound Obstet Gynecol, 21:277-282.

Jokubkiene L, Sladkevicius P, rovas L, Valentin L. (2006) Assessment of changes in endometrial and subendometrial volume and vascularity during the normal menstrual cycle using three-dimensional power Doppler ultrasound. Ultrasound Obstet Gynecol; 27: 672-9.

Jurkovic D, Geipel A, Gruboeck K, Jauniaux E, Natucci M, Campbell S. (1995) Three-dimensional ultrasound for the assessment of uterine anatomy and detection of congenital anomalies: a comparison with hysterosalpingography and two-dimensional sonography. Ultrasound Obstet Gynecol; 5 (4):233-7.

Kan AK, Abdalla HI, Gafar AH, Nappi L, Ogunyemi BO, Thomas A, et al (1999). Embryo transfer: ultrasound-guided versus clinical touch. Hum Reprod;14:1259-61.

Karande, V.C., Morris, R., Chapman, C., Rinehart, J. and Gleicher, N. (1999) Impact of the "physician factor" on pregnancy rates in a large assisted reproductive technology program: do too many cooks spoil the broth? Fertil. Steril., 71, 1001–1009.

Kepic, T, Applebaum, M. and Valle, J. (1992) Preovulatory follicular size, endometrial appearance, and estradiol levels in both con-ception and non-conception cycles: a retro-spective study. Presented at the 40th Annual Clinical Meeting of the American College of Obste-tricians and Gynecologists, April; Abstr. 20

Khalifa, E., Brzvski, R. G., Oehninger, S., Acosta, A. A. and Muasher, S.J. (1992) Sono-graphic appearance of the endometrium: the predictive value for the outcome of in vitro fertilization in stimulated cycles. Hum. Reprod.; 7, 677-80

Killick SR (2007). Ultrasound and receptivity of the endometrium. Reproductive BioMedicine Online: www.rbmonline.com/Article/2859; Vol 15 Mo 1; 63-67

Knutzen V, Stratton CJ, Sher G, McNamee PI, Huang TT, Soto- Albors C (1992). Mock embryo transfer in early luteal phase, the cycle before in vitro fertilization and embryo transfer a descriptive study. Fertil Steril;57:156- 162.

Kojima K, Nomiyama M, Kumamoto T, Matsumoto Y and Iwasaka T (2001) Transvaginal ultrasound-guided embryo transfer improves pregnancy and implantation rates after IVF. Hum Reprod16,2578–2582.

Kosmas IP, Janssens R, De Munck L, Al Turki H, Van der Elst J, Tournaye H. (2007) Ultrasound-guided embryo transfer does not offer any benefit in clinical outcome: a randomized controlled trial. Hum Reprod ; 22:1327-1334.

Krampl E, Zegermacher G, Eichler C, Obruca A, Strohmer H and Feichtinger W (1995) Air in the uterine cavity after embryo transfer. Fertil Steril 63, 366–370.

Krampl, E. and Feichtinger, W. (1993). Endo-metrial thickness and echo patterns [Letter]. Hum. Reprod., 8, 1339

Kunz G, Beil D, Deininger H, Wildt L, Leyendecker G. The dynamics of rapid sperm transport through the female genital track: evidence from vaginal sonography of uterine peristalsis and hysterosalpingoscintigraphy. Hum Reprod 1996;11:627- 632.

Kupesic S, Bekavac I, Bjelos D, Kurjak A. (2001) Assessment of endometrial receptivity by transvaginal color Doppler and three-dimensional power Doppler ultrasonography in patients undergoing in vitro fertilization procedures. J Ultrasound Med;20:125-34.

Kupesik S, Merce LT, Zodan T, Kurjak A. (2000) Normal and abnormal corpus luteum function. In Kupesic S, de Ziegler D, (Eds.): Ultrasound and Infertility. Lancs: The Parthenon Publishing Group,; 67-76.

Kyei-Mensah A, Maconochie N, Zaidi J, Pittrof R, Campbell S, Tan SL: (1996) Transvaginal three-dimensional ultrasound: reproducibility of ovarian and endometrial volume measurements. Fertil Steril, 66:718-722.

Lee A, Sator M, Kratochwil A, Deutinger J, Vytiska- Binsdorfer E, Bernaschek G. (1997) Endometrial volume change during spontaneous menstrual cycles: volumetry by transvaginal three-dimensional ultrasound. Fertil Steril; 68(5): 831-5.

Leeton J, Trounson A, Jessop D and Wood C (1982) The technique for human embryo transfer. Fertil Steril38,156–161.

Leibovitz Z, Grinin V, Rabia R, Degani S, Shapiro I, Tal J et al. (1999) Asseessement of endometrial receptivity for gestation in patients undergoing in vitro fertilization, using endometrial thickness and the endometrium-myometrium relative echogenicity coefficient. Ultrasound Obstet Gynecol; 14:194-9.

Leong M, Leung C, Tucker M, Wong C and Chan H (1986) Ultrasound-assisted embryo transfer. J in Vitro Fertil Embryo Transfer3,383–385.

Lesny P, Killick SR, Robinson J, Raven G, Maguiness SD (1999a). Embryo transfer and junctional zone contractions: is it safe to use a tenaculum? Hum Reprod; 14:2367-2370.

Lesny P, Killick SR, Robinson J, Titterington J, Maguiness SD (1999). Case report: ectopic pregnancy after transmyometrial embryo transfer. Fertil Steril;72:357 -359.

Lesny P, Killick SR, Tetlow RL, Manton DJ, Robinson J, Maguiness SD. (1999) Ultrasound evaluation of the uterine zonal anatomy during in-vitro fertilization and embryo transfer. Hum Reprod;14:1593–8.

Lesny P, Killick SR, Tetlow RL, Robinson J and Maguiness SD (1998) Embryo transfer—can we learn anything new from the observation of junctional zone contractions? Hum Reprod 13, 1540–1546.

Lesny P, Killick SR, Tetlow RL, Robinson J and Maguiness SD (1999) Embryo transfer and uterine junctional zone contractions. Hum Reprod Update5,87–88.

Lesny, P.L., Killick, S.R., Robinson, J. et al. (1999) Junctional zone contractions and embryo transfer: is it safe to use a tenaculum?. Hum. Reprod., 14, 2367–2370.

Letterie GS, Marshall L and Angle M (1999) A new coaxial catheter system with an echodense tip for ultrasonographically guided embryo transfer. Fertil Steril72,266–268.

Levi Setti PE, Albani E, Cavagna M, Bulletti C, Colombo GV and Negri L (2003) The impact of embryo transfer on implantation—a review. Placenta 24 (Suppl B), 20–26.

Lev-Toaff AS, Pinheiro LW, Bega G, Kurtz AB, Goldberg BB. (2001) Three-dimensional multiplanar sonohysterography: comparison with conventional twodimensional sonohysterography and X-ray hysterosalpingography. J Ultrasound Med; 20(4): 295-306.

Lewin A, Schenker JG, Avrech O, Shapira S, Safran A and Friedler S (1997) The role of uterine straightening by passive bladder distension before embryo transfer in IVF cycles. J Assist Reprod Genet14,32–34.

Li R, Lu L, Hao G, Zhong K, Cai Z, Wang W. (2005) Abdominal ultrasound-guided embryo transfer improves clinical pregnancy rates after in vitro fertilization: experiences from 330 clinical investigations. J Assist Reprod Genet; 22:3–8.

Li, T. C, Nutlall, L., Klentzeris, L. and Cooke, I. D. (1992). How well does ultrasonographic measurement of endometrial thickness predict the results of histological dating? Hum. Reprod.. 7, 1-5

Liedholm P, Sundstrom P and Wramsby H (1980) A model for experimental studies on human egg transfer. Arch Androl 5,92

Lindheim SR, Cohen MA and Sauer MV (1999) Ultrasound guided embryo transfer significantly improves pregnancy rates in women undergoing oocyte donation. Int J Gynaecol Obstet66,281–284.

Li-Wei Chien, M.D., Heng-Kien Au, M.D., Ping-Ling Chen, Ph.D., c Jean Xiao, M.D. and Chii-Ruey Tzeng, M.D. (2002) Assessment of uterine receptivity by the endometrial-subendometrial blood flow distribution pattern in women undergoing in vitro fertilization-embryo transfer. Fertil Steril; 78:245-251.

Lorusso F, Depalo R, Bettocchi S, Vacca M, Vimercati A, Selvaggi L.(2005) Outcome of in vitro fertilization after transabdominal ultrasound-assisted embryo transfer with a full or empty bladder. Fertil Steril ; 84:1046-104.

Mansour R, Aboulghar M, Serour G. (1990) Dummy embryo transfer: a technique that minimizes the problems of embryo transfer and improves the pregnancy rate in human in vitro fertilization. Fertil Steril. Oct; 54(4): 678-681.

Mansour RT and Aboulghar MA (2002) Optimizing the embryo transfer technique.Hum Reprod 17, 1149–1153.

Mansour RT, Aboulghar MA, Serour GI, Amin YM (1994). Dummy embryo transfer using methylene blue. Hum Reprod;9:1257–1259.

Mansour, R., Aboulghar, M. and Serour, G. (1990) Dummy embryo transfer: a technique that minimizes the problems of embryo transfer and improves the pregnancy rate in human in vitro fertilization. Fertil. Steril., 54, 678–681.

Martinez F, Coroleu B, Parriego M, Carreras O, Belil I, Parera N, Hereter L,Buxaderas R, Bar ri PN.(2001) Ultrasound-guided embryo transfer: immediate withdrawal of the catheter versus a 30 second wait. Hum Reprod ;16:871-874.

Matorras R, Urquijo E, Mendoza R, Corcostegui B, Exposito A and Rodriguez-Escudero FJ (2002) Ultrasound-guided embryo transfer improves pregnancy rates and increases the frequency of easy transfers. Hum Reprod 17,1762–1766.

McCarthy S, Scott G, Majumdar S, Shapiro B, Thompson S, Lange R, et al. (1989) Uterine junctional zone: MR study of water content and relaxation properties. Radiology;171:241–3.

Meldrum DR, Chetkowski R, Steingold KA, de Ziegler D, Cedars MI and Hamilton M (1987) Evolution of a highly successful in vitro fertilization embryo transfer program.Fertil Steril 64, 382–389.

Merce LT, Moreno C, Bau S. (1995) Assessment of luteal and periimplantation blood flow with color Doppler in AIH. In; abstract Book of ESHRE Symposium on Reproductive Medicina. Valencia, 9-11 march,; 12.

Merce LT. (2000) Doppler de los cambios ovaricos y endometriales preimplantatiorios. En Kurjak A, carrera JM, (Eds): Ecografia en Medicina Materno-Fetal. Barcelona: Masson; 87-104

Merce LT. (2000) studio Doppler de la implantacion y placentacion inicial. En Kurjak A, carrera JM, (Eds): Ecografia en Medicina Materno-Fetal. Barcelona: Masson,; 113-36.

Merce LT. Aplicationes del Doppler color en Reproduccion. (2002) IV Curso Teorico-Practico sobre Doppler en Ginecologia, Obstetrica y Ecocardiografia fetal. Barcelona, 2-4 de mayo,

Merce LT. Ultrasound markers of implantation. (2002). Ultrasound Rev Obstet Gynecol; 2:110-23

Merce LT. Ultrasound markers of implantation. In Kurjak A, Chervenak FA, (Eds.). (2004) Donald school Textbook of Ultrasound in Obsterics and Gynecology. New Delhi: Jaypee Brothers Medical Publishers,; pp 691-700

Merce TL, barco MJ, Bau S, Kurjak A (2008). Ultrasound Markers of implantation in Kurjak A, ChervenakFA (Eds): Donald School textbook of ultrasound in obstetrics and gynecology; New Delhi: JAYPEE Brothers Medical publishers LTD, 2008; 887-898.

Meriano, J., Weissman, A., Greenblaat, E.M., Ward, S. and Casper, R.F. (2000) The choice of embryo transfer catheter affects embryo implantation after IVF. Fertil. Steril.,74, 678–682.

Mirkin S, Jones EL, Mayer JF, Stadtmauer L, Gibbons WE and Oehninger S (2003) Impact of transabdominal ultrasound guidance on performance and outcome of transcervical uterine embryo transfer. J Assist Reprod Genet 20, 318–322.

Mitchell JD, Wardle PG, Foster PA and Hull MG (1989) Effect of bladder filling on embryo transfer. J in Vitro Fertil Embryo Transfer6,263–265.

Naaktgeboren N, Broers FC, Heijnsbroek I, Oudshoorn E, Verburg H and Van der Westerlaken L (1997) Hard to believe hardly discussed, nevertheless very important for the IVF/ICSI results: embryo transfer technique can double or halve the pregnancy rate.Hum Reprod 12 (Abstract Book 1), 149.

Naaktgeboren, N., Dieben, S., Heijnsbroek, I., Verburg, H. and Van der Westerlaken, L. (1998) Embryo transfer, easier said than done. Abstracts of the 16th World Congress on Fertility and Sterility and 54th Annual Meeting of the American Society for Reproductive Medicine, San Francisco, CA, USA, S352.

Nabi A, Awonuga A, Birch H, Barlow S and Stewart B (1997) Multiple attempts at embryo transfer: does this affect in-vitro fertilization treatment outcome? Hum Reprod12,1188–1190.

Nardo LG: (2005) Vascular endothelial growth factor expression in the endometrium during the menstrual cycle, implantation window and early pregnancy. Curr Opin Obstet Gynecol, 17:419-423.

Nazari A, Askari HA, Check JH and O, Shaughnessy A (1993) Embryo transfer technique as a cause of ectopic pregnancy in in-vitro fertilization. Fertil Steril 60, 919–921.

Ng EH, Chan CC, Tang OS, Yeung WS, Ho PC (2005). Endometrial and subendometrial blood flow measured by three-dimensional power Doppler ultrasound in patients with small intramural uterine fibroids during IVF treatment. Hum Reprod;20:501-506.

Ng EH, Chan CC, Tang OS, Yeung WS, Ho PC: (2006) The role of endometrial and subendometrial blood flows measured by three-dimensional power Doppler ultrasound in the prediction of pregnancy during IVF treatment. Hum Reprod, 21:164-170.

Ng EH, Chan CC, Tang OS, Yeung WS, Ho PC: (2006) The role of endometrial and subendometrial vascularity measured by three-dimensional power Doppler ultrasound in the prediction of pregnancy during frozen-thawed embryo transfer cycles. Hum Reprod, 21:1612-1617.

Ng EH, Yeung WS, Ho PC. (2009) Endometrial and sub endometrial vascularity are significantly lower in patients with endometrial volume 2.5 ml or less. Reprod Biomed Online;18:262-8.

Ng EHY, Chan CCW, Tang OS, Yeung WSB, Ho PC (2004). Endometrial and subendometrial blood flow measured during early luteal phase by three-dimensional power Doppler ultrasound in excessive ovarian responders. Human Reprod; 19: 924-31.

Ng EHY, Chan CCW, tang OS, Yeung WSB, Ho PC. (2004) Comparison of endometrial and subendometrial blood flow measured by three-dimensional power Doppler ultrasound between stimulated and natural cycles in the same patients. Hum Reprod; 19:2385-90.

Ng EHY, Chan CCW, tang OS, Yeung WSB, Ho PC. (2006) Factors affecting endometrial and subendometrial blood flow measured by three-dimensional power Doppler ultrasound during IVF treatment. Hum Reprod; 21: 1062-9

Nikas G, Develioglu OH, Toner JT. et al. (1999) Endometrial pinopodes indicate a shift in the window of receptivity in IVF cycles. Hum Reprod; 14:787-792.

Noyes N, Hapmton BS, Berkeley A, Licciardi F, Grifo J, Krey L. (2001) Factors useful in predicting the success of oocyte donation: a 3-year retrospective analysis. Fertil Steril; 76: 92-7.

Oliveira JB, Martins AM, Baruffi RL, Mauri AL, Petersen CG, Felipe V, Contart P, Pontes A and Franco Junior JG (2004) Increased implantation and pregnancy rates obtained by placing the tip of the transfer catheter in the central area of the endometrial cavity. Reprod Biomed Online 9,435–441.

Pairleitner H, Steiner H, Hasenoehrl G, Staudach A: (1999) Three-dimensional power Doppler sonography: imaging and quantifying blood flow and vascularization. Ultrasound Obstet Gynecol, 14:139-143.

Poindexter AN, Thompson DJ, Gibbons WE, Findley WE, Dodson MG, Young RL (1986). Residual embryos in failed embryo transfer. Fertil Steril;46:262- 267.

Pope CS, Cook EKD, Arny M, Novak A and Grow DR (2004) Influence of embryo transfer depth on in vitro fertilization and embryo transfer outcomes. Fertil Steril81,51–58.

Prapas Y, Prapas N, Hatziparasidou A, Prapa S, Nijs M, Vanderzwal-men P, et al. (1995) The echoguide embryo transfer maximizes the IVF results. Acta Eur Fertil;26:113–5.

Prapas Y, Prapas N, Hatziparasidou A, Vanderzwalmen P, Nijs M, Prapa S and Vlassis G (2001) Ultrasound-guided embryo transfer maximizes the IVF results on day 3 and day 4 embryo transfer but has no impact on day 5. Hum Reprod16,1904–1908.

Rabinowitz, R., Laufer, N., Lewin, A., Navot, D., Bar, I., Margalioth, E.J. and Schenker, J.J (1986). The value of ultrasonographic endome-trial measurement in the prediction of preg-nancy following in vitro fertilization. Fertil. Steril;, 45, 824-8

Raga F, Bonilla-Musoles F, Casan EM, Klein O, Bonilla F: (1999) Assessment of endometrial volume by three-dimensional ultrasound prior to embryo transfer: clues to endometrial receptivity. Hum Reprod, 14:2851-2854.

Raine –Fenning NJ, Campbel BK, Clewes JS, Johnson IR (2004). Endometrial and subendomtrial perfusion are impaired in women with unexplained subfertility. Hum Reprod; 19: 2605-2614.

Raine-Fenning N, Campbell B, Collier J, Brincat M, Johnson I: (2002) The reproducibility of endometrial volume acquisition and measurement with the VOCAL-imaging program. Ultrasound Obstet Gynecol, 19:69-75.

Raine-Fenning NJ, Campbell BK, Clewes JS, Johnson IR: (2003) The interobserver reliability of ovarian volume measurement is improved with three-dimensional ultrasound, but dependent upon technique. Ultrasound Med Biol b, 29:1685-1690.

Raine-Fenning NJ, Campbell BK, Clewes JS, Kendall NR, Johnson IR: (2003) The reliability of virtual organ computer-aided analysis (VOCAL) for the semiquantification of ovarian, endometrial and subendometrial perfusion. Ultrasound Obstet Gynecol a, 22:633-639.

Raine-Fenning NJ, Campbell BK, Kendall NR, Clewes JS, Johnson IR: (2004) Quantifying the changes in endometrial vascularity throughout the normal menstrual cycle with three-dimensional power Doppler angiography. Hum Reprod, 19:330-338.

Rashidi BH, Sadeghi M, Jafarabadi M, Tehrani Nejad ES. (2005) Relationships between pregnancy ratios following in vitro fertilization or intracytoplasmic sperm injection and endometrial thickness and pattern. Eur J Obstet Gynecol Reprod Biol; 2: 179-84.

Reine-Fenning N, Campbell BK, Clewes JS, Kendall NG, Johnson IR. (2004) Defining endometrial growth during the menstrual cycle with three-dimensional ultrasound. Br j Obstet Gynaecol; 111: 944-9.

Remohi J,Ardiles G, Garcia-Velasco JA, gaitan P, Simon C, Pellicer A. (1997) Endometrial thickness and serum oestradiol concentrations as predictors of outcome in oocyte donation. Hum Reprod; 12:2271-6

Riccabona M, Nelson TR, Pretorius DH. (1996) Three-dimensional ultrasound: accuracy of distance and volume measurements. Ultrasound Obstet Gynecol Jun; 7(6), 429-34.

Richter KS, Bugge KR, Bromer JG, Levy M. (2007) Relationship between endometrial thickness and embryo implantation, based on 1294 cycles of in vitro fertilization with transfer of two blastocyst-stage embryos. Fertil Steril; 1: 53-9.

Robert Z. Gergely, M.D.,Catherine Marin DeUgarte, M.D.,Hal Danzer, M.D.,Mark Surrey, M.D., David Hill, Ph.D. and Alan H. DeCherney, M.D. (2005) Three dimensional/four dimensional ultrasoundguided embryo transfer using the maximal implantation potential point. Fertility and Sterility 84: 500-503.

Roselund B, Sjöblom P and Hillensjö T (1996) Pregnancy outcome related to the site of embryo deposition in the uterus. J Assist Reprod Genet 13, 511–513.

Sallam HN and Sadek SS (2003) Ultrasound-guided embryo transfer: a meta-analysis of randomized controlled trials. Fertil Steril 80, 1042–1046.

Sallam HN, Agameya AF, Rahman AF, Ezzeldin F and Sallam AN (2002) Ultrasound measurement of the uterocervical angle before embryo transfer: a prospective controlled study. Hum Reprod 17,1767–1772.

Salle B, Bied-Damon V, Benchaib M, Desperes S, Gaucherand P, Rudigoz RC. (1998) Preliminary report of an ultrasonography and color Doppler uterine score to predict uterine receptivity in an in-vitro fer-tilization programme. Hum Reprod;13:1669–73.

Schild RL, Holthaus S, d'Alquen J, Fimmers R, Dorn C, van Der Ven H, Hansmann M: (2000) Quantitative assessment of subendometrial blood flow by three-dimensional-ultrasound is an important predictive factor of implantation in an in-vitro fertilization programme. Hum Reprod, 15:89-94.

Schild RL, Indefrei D, Eschweiler S, Van der Ven H, Fimmers R, Hansmann M: (1999) Three-dimensional endometrial volume calculation and pregnancy rate in an in-vitro fertilization programme. Hum Reprod, 14:1255-1258.

Schild RL, Knobloch C, Dorn C, Fimmers R, van der Ven H, Hansmann M: (2001) Endometrial receptivity in an in vitro fertilization program as assessed by spiral artery blood flow, endometrial thickness, endometrial volume, and uterine artery blood flow. Fertil Steril, 75:361-366.

Scholtes MCW, Wladimiroff JW, van Rijen HJM, Hop WCJ. (1989) Uterine and ovarian flow velocity waveforms in the normal menstrual cycle- a transvaginal study. Fertil Steril; 52:981-5.

Schoolcraft WB, Surrey ES and Gardner DK (2001) Embryo transfer: techniques and variables affecting success. Fertil Steril 76, 863–870.

Schulman JD (1986). Delayed expulsion of transfer fluid after IVF/ET. Lancet;1:44.

Scoutt LM, Flyn SD, Luthringer DJ, McCauley TR, McCarthy SM. (1991) Junctional zone of the uterus: correlation of MR imaging and histologic examination of hysterectomy specimens. Radiology;179:403–7.

Serafini, P., Batzofin, J., Nelson, and Olive, D. (1994). Sonographic uterine predictors of pregnancy in women undergoing ovulation induction for assisted reproductive treatments. Fertil. Steril, 62,815-22

Shaker AG, Fleming R, Jamieson ME, Yates RW, Coutts JR (1993). Assessment of embryo transfer after in-vitro fertilization: effects of glyceryl trinitrate. Hum Reprod;8:1426-1428.

Shamonki M, Schatman GL, Spandorfer SD and Rosenwaks Z (2005a) Ultrasound-guided embryo transfer may be beneficieal in preparation for an IVF cycle. Hum Reprod 20 (10),2844-49.

Shamonki MI, Spandorfer SD and Rosenwaks Z (2005b) Ultrasound-guided embryo transfer and the accuracy of trial embryo transfer. Hum Reprod 20(3),709–716.

Sharif K, Afnan M, Lenton W. Mock (1995) Embryo transfer with a full bladder immediately before the real transfer for in-vitro fertilization treatment: the Birmingham experience of 113 cases. Hum Reprod. Jul; 10(7): 1715-1718.

Sher G, Dodge S, Maassarani G, Knutzen V, Zouves C, Feinman M. (1993) Management of suboptimal sonographic endometrial patterns in pa-tients undergoing in-vitro fertilization and embryo transfer. Hum Re-prod;8:347–9.

Sher, G., Herbert, C, Maassarani, G. and Jacobs, M. H. (1991) Assessment of the late proliferative phase endometrium by ultra-sonography in patients undergoing in vitro fer-tilization and embryo transfer (IVF/ET). Hum. Reprod.; 6, 232-7

Sherer DM, Abulafia O: (2001) Angiogenesis during implantation, and placental and early embryonic development. Placenta, 22:1-13.

Sladkevicius P, Valentin L, Marsal K. (1993) Blood flow velocity in the uterine and ovarian arteries during the normal menstrual cycle. Ultrasound Obstet Gynecol; 3: 199-208.

Smith, B., Porter, R., Ahuja, K. and Craft, I. (1984) Ultrasonic assessment of endometrial changes in stimulated cycles in an in vitro fertil-ization and embryo transfer program. J. In Vitro Fertil. Embryo Transfer, 1, 233-8

Steer, C V., Tan, S. L., Mason, B. A. and Campbell, S. (1994) Midluteal-phasc vaginal color Doppler assessment of uterine artery impedance in a subfertile population. Fertil. Steril; 61, 53-8

Steer, C. V., Campbell, S., Tan, S. L., Cravford, T, Mills, C, Mason, B. A. and Collins,' W. P. (1992). The use of transvaginal color flow imaging after in vitro fertilization to identify optimum uterine conditions before embryo transfer. Fertil. Steril; 57, 372-6

Steptoe, P.C. and Edwards, R. (1976) Reimplantation of a human embryo with subsequent tubal pregnancy. Lancet, 1, 880 -882.

Sterzik, K., Grab, D., Sasse, V., Hutter, W., Rosenbusch, B. and Terinde, R. (1989) Doppler sonographic findings and their corre-lation with implantation in an in vitro fertiliza-tion program. Fertil. Steril; 52, 825-8

Strickler RC, Christianson C, Crane JP, Curato A, Knight AB and Yang V (1985) Ultrasound guidance for human embryo transfer. Fertil Steril 43, 54–61.

Sundstrom P, Wramsby H, Persson PH and Liedholm P (1984) Filled bladder simplifies human embryo transfer. Br J Obstet Gynaecol91,506–507.

Sundtsrom P. (1998) Establishment of a successful pregnancy following in-vitro fertilization with an endometrial thickness of on more than 4mm. Hum Reprod; 13:1550-2

Tan SL, Biljan MM. (2000) Selection of candidates for in vitro fertilization based on color Doppler findings. In Kupesic S, De Ziegler D, (Eds): Ultrasound and Infertility. London: the Prathenon Publishing Group; 155-68

Tan SL, zaidi J, Campbell S, Doyle P, Collins W. (1996) Blood flow changes in the ovarian and uterine arteries during the normal menstrual cycle. Am j obstet Gynecol; 175:625-31

Tang B, Gurpide E. (1993) Direct effect of gonadotropins on decidualization of human endometrial stroma cells. J Steroid Biochem Mol Biol; 47:115-21

Tang OS, Ng EHY, So WWK and Ho PC (2001) Ultrasound-guided embryo transfer: a prospective randomized controlled trial. Hum Reprod16,2310–2315.

Tekay A, Martikainen H, Jouppila P. (1996) The clinical value of transvaginal color Doppler ultrasound in assisted reproductive technology proce-dures. Hum Reprod;11:1589–91.

Tekay A, Martikainen H, Jouppila P: (1995) Blood flow changes in uterine and ovarian vasculature, and predictive value of transvaginal pulsed color Doppler ultrasonography in an in-vitro fertilization programme. Hum Reprod, 10:688-693.

Tetlow RL, Richmond I, Manton DJ, Greenman J, Turnbull LW, Killick SR. (1999) Histological analysis of the uterine junctional zone as seen by transvaginal ultrasound. Ultrasound Obstet Gynecol;14:188- 93.

Tsai HD, Chang CC, Hsieh YY, Lee CC, Lo HY. (2000) Artificial insemination. Role of endometrial thickness and pattern, of vascular impedance of the spiral and uterine arteries, and of the dominant follicle. J Reprod Med; 3: 195-200.

Turnbull LW, Manton JD, Horsman A, Killick SR. (1995) Magnetic resonance imaging changes in uterine zonal anatomy during a conception cycle. Br J Obstet Gynaecol;102:330–1.

Van de Pas MMC, Weima S, Looman CWN and Broekmans FJM (2003) The use of fixed distance embryo transfer after IVF/ICSI equalizes the success rates among physicians. Hum Reprod 18, 774–780.

Visser, D.S., Fouri, F.L. and Kruger, H.F. (1993) Multiple attempts at embryo transfer: effect on pregnancy outcome in an in vitro fertilization and embryo transfer program. J. Assist. Reprod. Genet., 10, 37–43.

Waterstone, J., Curson, R. and Parsons, J. (1991) Embryo transfer to low uterine cavity. Lancet, 337, 1413.

Weissman A, Gotlieb L, Casper RF. (1999) The detrimental effect of increased endometrial thickness on implantation and pregnancy ratios and outcome in an in vitro fertilization program. Fertil Steril; 1: 147-9.

Welker, B. G., Gembruch, U., Diedrich, K., al-Hasani, S. and Krebs, D. (1989) Transvagi-nal sonography of the endometrium during ovum pick-up in stimulated cycles for in vitro fertilization./. Ultrasound Med , 8, 549-53

Wisanto A, Janssens R, Deschacht J, Camus M, Devroey P, Van Steirteghem AC. (1989) Performance of different embryo transfer catheters in a human in vitro fertilization program. Fertil Steril. Jul; 52(1): 79-84.

Wood C, McMaster R, Rennie G, Trounson A and Leeton J (1985) Factors influencing pregnancy rates following in vitro fertilization and embryo transfer. Fertil Steril 43,245–250.

Wood EG, Batzer FR, Go KJ, Gutmann JN, Corson SL. (2000) Ultrasound-guided soft catheter embryo transfers will improve pregnancy rates in in-vitro fertilization. Hum Reprod. Jan; 15(1): 107-112.

Woolcott R and Stanger J (1997) Potentially important variables identified by transvaginal ultrasound-guided embryo transfer. Hum Reprod 12, 963–966.

Woolcott R, Stanger J (1998). Ultrasound tracking of the movement of embryo-associated air bubbles on standing after transfer. Hum Reprod;13:2107-9.

Wu HM, Chiang CH, Huang HY, Chao AS, Wang HS, Soong YK: (2003) Detection of the subendometrial vascularization flow index by three-dimensional ultrasound may be useful for predicting the pregnancy rate for patients undergoing in vitro fertilization- embryo transfer. Fertil Steril, 79:507-511.

Yaman C, Ebner T, Sommergruber M, Polz W, Tews G. (2000) Role of three-dimensional ultrasonographic measurement of endometrium volume as a predictor of pregnancy outcome in an IVF-ET program: a preliminary study. Fertil Steril; 74(4): 797-801.

Yaman C, Jesacher k, Polz W: (2003) Accuracy of three-dimensional transvaginal ultrasound in uterus volume measurements: comparison with two-dimensional ultrasound. Ultrasound Med boil; 29;1681-1684

Yaman C, Sommergruber M, Ebner T, Polz W, Moser M, Tews G: (1999) Reproducibility of transvaginal three-dimensional endometrial volume measurements during ovarian stimulation. Hum Reprod, 14:2604-2608.

Yang J-H, Wu M-Y, Chen C-D, Jiang M-C, Ho H-N, yang Y-S. (1999) Association of endometrial blood flow as determined by a modified color Doppler technique with subsequent outcome of in-vitro fertilization. Hum reprod; 14;1606-10.

Yuval Y, Liptz S, Dor J, Achiron R. (1999) The relationship between endometrial thickness, and blood flow and pregnancy rates in in-vitro fertilization. Human Reprod; 14:1967-71

Zaidi J, Campbell S, Pittrof R, tan SL. (1995) Endometrial thickness, morphology, vascular penetration and velocimetry in predicting implantation in an in vitro fertilization program. Ultrasound Obstet Gynecol; 6; 191-8

Zaidi, J., Pittrof, R., Shaker, A, Kyei-Mensah, A., Campbell, S. and Tan, S. L. (1996) Assessment of uterine artery blood flow on the day of human chorionic gonadotropin administration by transvaginal color Doppler ultrasound in an in vitro fertilization program. Fertil. Steril; 65,377-81

Zech, H., Stecher, A., Riedler, I. et al. (1997) High implantation rate with a fast and atraumatic embryo transfer technique. Hum. Reprod., 12 (Abstract Bk 1), p. 156

Zhang X, Chen CH, Confino E, Barnes R, Milad M, Kazer RR. (2005) Increased endometrial thickness is associated with improved treatment outcome for selected patients undergoing in vitro fertilization-embryo transfer. Fertil Steril; 2: 336-40.

Zollner U, Zollner KP, Specketer MT, Blissing S, Muller T, Steck T, Dietl J: (2003) Endometrial volume as assessed by three dimensional ultrasound is a predictor of pregnancy outcome after in vitro fertilization and embryo transfer. Fertil Steril; 80:1515-1517.

Zouves C, Erenus M, Gomel V (1991). Tubal ectopic pregnancy after in vitro fertilization and embryo transfer: a role for proximal occlusion or salpingectomy after failed distal tubal surgery. Fertil Steril;56: 691–695.

Part 2

Innovative Laboratory Aspects of IVF, Present and Future Techniques

4

Methods for Sperm Selection for In Vitro Fertilization

Nicolás M. Ortega and Pablo Bosch
Departamento de Biología Molecular,
Facultad de Ciencias Exactas Fco-Qcas y Naturales,
Universidad Nacional de Río Cuarto, Río Cuarto,
Córdoba y Consejo Nacional de Investigaciones Científicas y Tecnológicas (CONICET),
Argentina

1. Introduction

The outcome of assisted reproductive technologies (ARTs) depends mostly on the quality of input material (oocytes and sperm) used in these procedures. The number of transferable embryos produced in these programs depends on both provision of high quality mature oocytes and adequate numbers of good quality spermatozoa capable of supporting embryo development to term. Semen samples are cellular mixtures composed of: precursor germ cells, subpopulations of viable and nonviable spermatozoa, variable amounts of debris, and multiple leukocyte subtypes, all suspended in seminal plasma (SP). Based on these characteristics and the heterogeneity of the sperm population within the ejaculate, several separation techniques such as swim-up and density gradients (e.g. Percoll®) have been developed. These techniques not only allow for selection of sperm with enhanced motility but may also be used to remove the extender and dead cells (up 50% of total) present in frozen-thawed sperm samples. In addition, selection of normal spermatozoa is of upmost importance in cases of male infertility caused by semen deficiencies characterized by teratospermia, asthenozoospermia and/or oligospermia.

The ideal protocol for enrichment/selection of sperm cells with high fertilizing ability should be: a) non-toxic for spermatozoa, b) easy to perform and inexpensive, c) able to support high-throughput sample processing, d) capable of selecting the best sperm subpopulation for ARTs, leaving behind, seminal plasma, extender (in case of frozen semen) and bioactive substances and cells (leukocytes) that could damage sperm cells. Despite the efforts invested in developing an ideal sperm selection technique by laboratories around the word, to date no single sperm selection protocol meets all desirable characteristics mentioned above. Today, it is recognized that the sperm is more than a mere DNA delivery vehicle to the oocyte; there is evidence that these highly specialized cells play a role far beyond the fertilization process by contributing paternal mRNAs, which it is believed to be crucial for normal early and late embryonic development (Barroso et al., 2009). Therefore, development of systems that allow for identifying the best spermatozoa for fertilization would contribute to improve the currently low live birth rates achieved by ARTs (Wright et al., 2008).

Most sperm selection protocols in use today for ARTs fall in one of the following categories: sperm migration, filtration, density gradient centrifugation or a combination of these methods. During the decision-making process to select a sperm separation protocol is important to consider both the type of infertility and the particular assisted reproductive approach to be used to treat it. For instance, high sperm numbers with vigorous motility are required for successful intrauterine insemination. On the other hand, few motile sperm cells, in the order of thousands, are required for conventional IVF, and even fewer to perform ICSI.

It has been well documented in all mammal species studied so far that ejaculated spermatozoa are subjected to a natural-occurring sperm selection process in the female reproductive tract in order to maximize the chances of successful reproduction. This differential sperm transport favors the ascent of morphologically normal spermatozoa with enhanced fertilizing ability. These natural barriers encountered by spermatozoa in vivo are partially or completely absent when ARTs are applied. Therefore, there is real concern about the possibility of using spermatozoa with suboptimal fertilization and embryo development potential. This is especially true during ICSI in which a single spermatozoon is selected by the technician based solely on motility and morphology parameters. Experimental data indicate that normal sperm morphology is not necessarily associated with DNA integrity (Avendano & Oehninger, 2011) what raises concerns about potential transmission of DNA alterations to next generations.

Knowledge from the natural sperm selection mechanisms that occur in vivo and insights from research in the area of the molecular mechanism that govern sperm physiology will provide basic information for improving current methods of sperm selection and developing novel procedures for accurately select the best spermatozoa for ARTs. In particular, the development of technologies in which a spermatozoon is mechanically introduced by the embryologist into the oocyte, bypassing all natural barriers for sperm selection, emphasize the need for more accurate sperm markers of fertilizing and normal developmental potential.

In the first section of this review we will describe the principles and discuss advantages and disadvantages of established sperm selection methodologies currently in use in the clinical setting. In the second part of this chapter, we will introduce advanced sperm selection techniques and emerging approaches to enrich sperm samples for ARTs.

2. Sperm selection techniques

2.1 Sperm washing

Sperm washing is a simple method which involves the centrifugation of the semen sample once or twice in order to pellet the sperm cells and remove the seminal plasma. The pellet is resuspended in appropriate media and used for ARTs (Bjorndahl et al., 2005; Edwards et al., 1969; Lopata et al., 1978). One of the major disadvantages of this method for sperm preparation is the oxidative cell damage caused by reactive oxygen species (ROS) generated in packaged cells after centrifugation. Sperm plasma membrane contains high amounts of poly-unsaturated fatty acids which are highly susceptible to lipid peroxidation by ROS. Consequently, SP provides ROS metabolizing enzymes and small molecular mass, free radical scavengers such as vitamin C and uric acid to protect germinal cells from damage.

Therefore, sperm function and DNA integrity can be compromised when SP is removed from the ejaculate.

Although centrifugation is useful to remove the SP, the overall sperm quality, in terms of motility remains unaltered or reduced since both motile and immotile fractions of sperm cells are subjected to the gravitational force, with the associated risk of removing part of the motile fraction with the supernatant that is discarded. In addition, centrifugation has been reported to be responsible for chromatin damage in human and stallion spermatozoa (Edwards et al., 1969; Morrell et al., 2011; Mortimer, 2000).

Despite numerous drawbacks associated with this approach, sperm washing is routinely used in the livestock industry to remove most of SP prior to adding the extender for cryopreservation. Extenders for animal semen such as milk- or egg yolk-based extenders, typically contain antioxidants which may counteract oxidant metabolites released during the procedure (Morrell et al., 2011).

2.2 Sperm migration

Mahadevan & Baker (1984) developed the classical washing swim-up (WSU) method, which is easy to perform and very cost effective. It is based on spermatozoa self-propelled active movement from a single centrifuged, pre-washed cell pellet, into an overlaying medium which serves as a hospitable environment for healthy sperm. Normal spermatozoa move away from seminal plasma, but those with tail abnormalities are not capable of migrating into the swim-up medium. Only a small fraction of total motile sperm is recovered by the WSU methodology, therefore its use is mostly restricted to ejaculates with high sperm counts and good motility (Mahadevan & Baker, 1984). The WSU is currently the standard technique used in IVF laboratories for patients with normozoospermia and female infertility. Since WSU includes a centrifugation step, it raises concern about the possibility of sperm plasma membrane and DNA damage due to ROS buildup from pelleted sperm cells, debris and leukocytes (Ford, 1990). To reduce ROS generation and the consequent damage to sperm cells, a modification of the classic WSU procedure was introduced. In this alternative swim-up procedure the liquefied semen sample is directly subjected to swim-up avoiding the initial centrifugation step. Here, sperm population is either underneath, on top or to one side of the migration medium (Mortimer, 2000). Some studies show significantly better midpiece and tail morphology after swim-up than after washing (Hallap et al., 2004).

It has also been shown that swim-up directly from semen into a migration medium supplemented with highly purified hyaluronic acid (HA) favors the selection of motile sperm with intact membranes, resulting in a higher pregnancy rate in clinical IVF programs (Jakab et al., 2005; Wikland et al., 1987).

Side migration is another technique based on the sperm ability to selectively move from one point to another (Hinting & Lunardhi, 2001). Unlike swim-up in which sperm cells move upwards into the medium, in the side migration technique (SMT) sperm move horizontally leaving behind immotile spermatozoa, round cells and debris. According to Hinting & Lunardhi (2001), SMT is an effective and physiological approach to obtain sperm for ICSI from poor-quality semen samples. In their study, semen from men affected with oligozoospermia (sperm concentrations of less than 20 million spermatozoa/ml) were subjected to side migration. The subpopulation of spermatozoa recovered had better morphology, viability, membrane integrity and nuclear chromatin integrity compared with those selected by traditional WSU and Percoll® gradient columns (PGC) (Hinting & Lunardhi, 2001). However, the number of sperm recovered is low, what limits the use of this technique to select sperm for ICSI procedures.

2.3 Sperm sedimentation

Tea et al. (1984) developed a very gentle separation method which combines swim-up from liquefied semen with a sedimentation step. The sperm selection is accomplished by using a special glass or plastic tube with an inner cone, design that allows for only those spermatozoa capable of swimming out from the liquidized semen to sediment in the inner cone. Since no centrifugation steps are required, generation of ROS is minimized and so is the sperm damage, rendering a very clean fraction of highly motile spermatozoa. The main disadvantage of this method is the very low recovery rate which makes it unpractical for intrauterine insemination or IVF.

2.4 Filtration

Glass wool filtration is a very simple, but more expensive procedure, which yields a higher total number of motile spermatozoa compared with those in the swim-up or migration centrifugation protocol, since the whole volume of the ejaculate can be filtrated. This method is also effective at eliminating leukocytes and cell debris, reducing ROS production and ROS-induced sperm damage (Henkel et al., 2005). A major advantage of this approach is that it selects normally chromatin-condensed spermatozoa, a parameter considered as predictive of fertilization ability in vitro.

Motile and viable spermatozoa from poor-quality semen can be recovered using a column of glass beads. This procedure is quick and simple and results in enrichment of the population of spermatozoa of interest. Due to the high sperm recovery, glass filtration method is especially useful for intrauterine insemination. Unluckily, the potential risk of glass bead spilling over into the insemination media has precluded its widespread use in ARTs. An alternative filtration method uses columns of Sephadex beads to produce high yields of morphologically normal sperm cells.

2.5 Density gradient centrifugation

In this procedure, diluted semen is placed on top of a conical centrifuge tube containing increasingly dense layers of a liquid solution called density medium. In the standard procedure for sperm preparation two layers of density medium are used. After centrifuging, highly motile sperm cells are enriched in the soft pellet at the bottom of the tube. The recovered sperm pellet is then washed by centrifugation to remove the density medium. Sperm damage during density gradient selection has been attributed to ROS accumulation associated with multiple centrifugation steps.

Polyvinylpyrrolidone (PVP)-coated silica particles (Percoll®) has been extensively used as a density medium to prepare fresh or frozen sperm specimens for human and animal ARTs. Vast experimental and clinical data support the effectiveness of the Percoll-based gradient methodology to produce viable, highly motile, morphologically normal populations of spermatozoa for intrauterine insemination, gamete intrafallopian transfer, and conventional IVF and ICSI (Moohan & Lindsay, 1995). Studies that compared WSU with density gradient procedure indicated that the latter is capable of yielding sperm populations with higher percentages of morphologically normal forms and nuclear integrity (Sakkas et al., 2000; Tomlinson et al., 2001). However, exposure of sperm to Percoll® can damage sperm membranes and there exists the risk of contamination of Percoll® with endotoxins, which in turn can cause an inflammatory response in the female reproductive tract. This led to the withdrawal of Percoll® from the market for clinical use in human ARTs in 1996 (Henkel & Schill, 2003).

Alternative commercial density gradients have been developed and are commonly used in human assisted reproduction: Nycodenz® (Nyegaard & Co., Oslo, Norway), PureSperm® (NidaCon Laboratories AB, Gothenburg, Sweden), IxaPrep® (MediCult, Copenhagen, Denmark), SilSelect® (FertiPro N.V., Beernem, Belgium), and ISolate® (Irvine Scientific, Santa Ana, CA, USA). Among these, PureSperm® IxaPrep®, SilSelect®, and ISolate® are silane-coated products which have been promoted as being safer than the PVP-coated particles (Percoll®). These products are non-irritating and have been approved for human in vivo use as they are all bioassay endotoxin-tested and easy to wash out.

2.6 Advanced and emerging sperm separation techniques

In this section we introduce advanced sperm separation/selection procedures. Based on the main criteria used to select a sperm subpopulation, these procedures can be classified as: selection by differential sperm surface charge (electrophoretic separation and Zeta potential), selection of non-apoptotic spermatozoa (magnetic-activated cell sorting), selection based on the sperm membrane maturity (hyialuronic-acid sperm binding) and selection based on ultramorphologic criteria (real-time motile sperm organelle morphology examination -MSOME-, intracytoplasmic morphologically selected sperm injection -IMSI- and ICSI using polarization microscopy). Each advanced methodology has been subjected to prospective studies to determine its ability to affect sperm quality, fertility rate and clinical pregnancy rates. In general, application of these procedures have improved assisted reproductive technology (ART) outcomes, however, to date the number of clinical trials are insufficient to draw definitive conclusions.

Finally, we will comment on emerging approaches for sperm selection which are currently in a developmental phase. These include: Raman spectroscopy, confocal light absorption and scattering microscopy -CLASS- and sperm chemotactic-based methods.

2.6.1 Sperm surface charge for sperm selection

There are two different approaches to select sperm based on the differential net electric charge on the sperm plasma membrane: electrophoretic system (SpermSep® CS-10, NuSep Ltd., Frenchs Forest, Australia) (Ainsworth et al., 2005) and zeta potential method (Chan et al., 2006).

2.6.1.1 Electrophoretic system

The electrophoresis-based technology was developed at Dr. Aitken´s laboratory in Australia (Ainsworth et al., 2005) and later commercialized by NuSep Ltd. as Microflow® CS-10 (renamed to SpermSep® CS-10). This device uses an electric field to separate sperm cells based on size and electronegative charge. It is composed of four chambers: two outer chambers and two inner chambers (incubation and collection). The outer chambers (filled with buffer) house the platinum-coated titanium mesh electrodes. A polyacrilamyne membrane separates the outer chambers from the inner chambers allowing for the movement of small molecules, water and ions between them. The inner chambers comprise the inoculation compartment and the collection compartment separated by a polycarbonate separation membrane which pore size excludes leukocytes and precursor germ cells that normally contaminate semen samples. The semen specimen is loaded into the incubation chamber and allowed to equilibrate for 5 min before applying a current of 75 mA and variable voltage (18-21 V). The selected sperm subpopulation is recovered from the collection chamber after 5 min of application of the electric field and it is ready for ARTs.

There is evidence that the electronegativity on the sperm surface indicates normal differentiation and is associated with CD52 expression on sperm membrane (Schroter et al., 1999) and other glycoproteins (Ainsworth et al., 2011). These observations and the fact that CD52 is correlated with normal sperm morphology and capacitation (Giuliani et al., 2004), may account for the ability of the electrophoresis separation method to select sperm with significantly improved morphology with low levels of DNA damage (Ainsworth et al., 2005). Key futures of the electrophoresis system that make it attractive for ART laboratories are: the whole process of selection can take only a few minutes and the generation of ROS is minimized because of lack of centrifugation steps. On the other hand, the cost associated with acquisition of the electrophoresis separation device may be prohibitive for andrology laboratories with limited resources.

The first live birth from an embryo conceived with a spermatozoon selected by the novel electrophoretic approach was reported in 2007 (Ainsworth et al., 2007). The study involved a couple with long-term infertility associated with extensive sperm DNA damage. Later, a prospective controlled trial was performed to demonstrate that the membrane-based electrophoresis system is as effective as and considerably faster than the DGC to prepare spermatozoa for both IVF and ICSI (Fleming et al., 2008).

2.6.1.2 Zeta potential method

Sperm cells can be selected based on their negative zeta electrokinetic potential (Chan et al., 2006) which is the overall charge a particle, in this particular case a spermatozoon, acquires in a specific medium. A mature sperm cell has a negative zeta potential of -16 to -20 mV (differential potential between the sperm membrane and its surroundings) (Ishijima et al., 1991). The zeta potential method is very simple to perform and it does not require special equipment, therefore it is inexpensive. Briefly, washed sperm in serum-free medium is introduced in a conical tube which has been positively charged by rubbing or rotating the tube on a latex glove. Electronegatively charged sperm (mature) attach to the walls of the tube by electrostatic forces and the non-adherent sperm fraction and other contaminants are removed by inverting the tube. Selected adherent sperm cells are recovered by rinsing the tube with serum-supplemented medium.

Regarding the morphology and functional characteristics of sperm selected by zeta potential, experimental data indicated that this method advantages the conventional DGC in terms of percentage of morphologically normal sperm, hyperactivation, DNA integrity and maturity, but not motility (Chan et al., 2006). Results from a randomized prospective study with sperm selected with a combination of DGC/zeta potential or DGC alone previous to ICSI indicated that the combination may increase fertilization rates and possibly pregnancy rates in infertile couples associated with male factor infertility (Kheirollahi-Kouhestani et al., 2009). However, definitive data that demonstrate the benefits of applying the zeta potential approach to select sperm for human assisted conception is still missing.

2.6.2 Selection of non-apoptotic spermatozoa

2.6.2.1 Magnetic-activated cell sorting (MACS)

The externalization of the phospholipid phosphatidylserine (PS) to the sperm plasma membrane is a characteristic feature of the apoptotic phenomenon that occurs early during the process of sperm cell death. This basic knowledge has prompted investigators to develop a magnetic-based selection system for sperm cells that can separate early apoptotic from non-apoptotic germ cells (MACS, Miltenyi Biotec GmbH, Bergisch Gladbach, Germany). Since externalized PS has high affinity to Annexin V, apoptotic sperm cells bind to Annexin V-conjugated paramagnetic microbeads. The magnetically labeled sample is passed through a magnetic column where magnetically labeled apoptotic or dead spermatozoa are retained in the column while the unlabeled non-apoptotic spermatozoa are collected in the flow-through for further processing for ARTs (Grunewald et al., 2001; Manz et al., 1995).

Despite magnetic cell sorting method is highly effective at removing apoptotic sperm cells, unfortunately it is not able to eliminate leukocytes, immature germ cells, seminal plasma and other contaminants from the semen sample. This is the reason why MACS separation is normally performed in conjunction with DGC (Said et al., 2005a; Said et al., 2005b). Repeated centrifugations and resuspensions associated with DGC can cause sperm loses imposing a limitation for semen samples characterized by limited sperm counts (Said et al., 2008).

Non-apoptotic markers in the MACS-selected population such as high mitochondrial potential and low caspase activation are consistent with the known selection criterion of this methodology. In addition, sperm sample parameters that are improved in the subpopulation selected by MACS include: sperm motility and morphology, sperm DNA damage and hamster oocyte penetration potential of spermatozoa (Lee et al., 2010; Said et al., 2006a; Said et al., 2006b). Clinical pregnancy data collected so far indicate that the use of MACS may be of especial value for cases of male infertility associated with high incidence of apoptotic and DNA damaged sperm (Dirican et al., 2008).

2.6.3 Selection based on sperm membrane maturity

2.6.3.1 Hyaluronic acid sperm binding

The presence of HA binding sites on sperm outer membrane is regarded as a sign of sperm maturity, and constitutes the basic principle for a sperm binding assay (Jakab et al., 2005). In this assay, HA is immobilized on a solid surface (polystyrene culture dish) and the washed sperm sample is allowed to interact with the HA coated surface for 15 min. An individual sperm attached to the dish is picked up with the ICSI pipette and used for oocyte injection.

As HA is a natural occurring compound present in cervical mucus, cumulus cells and follicular fluid, the binding method is considered to have minimal biosafety risks for both the embryo and the patient.

The device called PICSI® (preselected intracytoplasmatical sperm injection), commercialized by ORIGIO MidAtlantic Devices Inc. (Mt Laurel, NJ, USA), uses a conventional polystyrene culture dish enhanced with tree microdots of hyaluronan where the sperm suspension is added.

Sperm maturity has been associated with certain desirable sperm traits such as: improved viability and motility, intact acrosomes, lower caspase-3 activation and lower frequency of chromosomal aneuploidies (Huszar et al., 2007; Huszar et al., 2003). Studies documenting the use of sperm selected by HA method in the clinical ART setting are still scarce and somehow contradictory. While one study reported significantly increased fertilization rate of oocytes injected with HA-selected sperm and only a marginal effect on pregnancy rate (Nasr-Esfahani et al., 2008), in other studies by Permegiani et al. (2010a; 2010b) oocytes injected with sperm selected by the binding method originated better quality embryos but no effect was detected on fertilization and pregnancy rates.

2.6.4 Selection based on live sperm morphology

It has been long recognized that sperm morphology is one of the major determinants of male fertility both in vitro and in vivo. ICSI is an assisted reproductive technique that is gaining acceptance for treatment of different forms of male infertility. In this procedure, a sperm cell is selected by the embryologist based on sperm morphology and motility and introduced into the mature oocyte, bypassing all natural selection barriers at fertilization. However, sperm evaluation at x 400 magnification (which is the standard magnification used to select sperm for ICSI) is unable to provide enough resolution for an accurate sperm morphological assessment.

With the objective of improving accuracy of sperm selection based on morphological features, Bartoov et al. (2002) developed a method for real-time sperm evaluation known as motile sperm organelle morphology examination (MSOME). MSOME sperm evaluation is performed in an inverted light microscope equipped with high-power differential interference contrast optics (Nomarski/DIC; magnification x150) enhanced by digital imaging (magnification, ×44) to achieve a total magnification of over 6000. At this magnification, it is possible to define the morphological normalcy of five sperm organelles (acrosome, postacrosomal lamina, neck, tail and nucleus) as observed at high magnification. Among these organelles, evaluation of sperm nucleus (shape and chromatin content) by MSOME appears be the most important feature conditioning ICSI outcome (Bartoov et al., 2003). Intracytoplasmic morphologically selected sperm injection (IMSI) is a modification of ICSI, in which the injected spermatozoon is selected by the technician at high magnification using MSOME normalcy criteria. When these techniques are used correctly by trained personnel, a significant correlation between morphology and fertilization rate was demonstrated (Bartoov et al., 2002). In addition, pregnancy and live birth rates were significantly higher in the IMSI group compared with that in the conventional ICSI group, but IMSI failed to boost fertilization and cleavage rates and did not improve embryo morphology. Similarly, Souza Setti et al. (2010) reported that IMSI improved pregnancy and abortion rates, but not fertilization rate. In conjunction, these results suggest that the sperm morphology traits that guide sperm selection during IMSI will have repercussions in late ART outcomes as evidenced by increased pregnancy and birth rates and diminished abortion rates.

Another optical system used to select live sperm for ICSI is based on birefringency (Gianaroli et al., 2008) generated by the incidence of polarized light on longitudinally oriented protein filaments on the postacrosomal region of the sperm (Baccetti, 2004). Sperm birefringency is evaluated with an inverted microscope equipped with polarizing and analyzing lenses. The proportion of birefringent sperm in a sample is correlated positively with sperm concentration, motility and viability (Gianaroli et al., 2008). In addition, using this optical system, it is possible to differentiate acrosome-reacted from acrosome-intact sperm before microinjection. It has been hypothesized that microinjection of acrosome reacted sperm during ICSI would improve the outcomes of this technique since it mimics more closely the natural phenomenon of fertilization. Clinical data collected so far support this hypothesis, as pregnancy rates originated from embryos produced with acrosome-reacted spermatozoa were significantly higher compared with those in the control group (ICSI with non-reacted spermatozoa) (Gianaroli et al., 2010).

2.6.5 Emerging methods for sperm selection

2.6.5.1 Raman spectroscopy

It has been documented that sperm cells with apparently normal morphology may have DNA fragmentation and other types of DNA damage (Angelopoulos et al., 1998; Avendano et al., 2009), which can affect embryo quality and pregnancy outcome if ICSI is performed with such defective sperm cells (Avendano et al., 2010). In light of the worldwide use of ICSI as major tool to treat infertility, the development of a technique that can non-invasively provide information about sperm chromatin packaging and nuclear normalcy before sperm injection would impact positively on ART outcomes. Micro-Raman spectroscopy holds promise to provide information about packaging of nuclear DNA in individual living sperm cells. Raman spectroscopy is a spectroscopic technique that examines the inelastic scattering of photons (a change in frequency of photons) caused by molecular bonds. The photons originated from a laser source are absorbed by the sample and then reemitted with a frequency different to that in the original source what is called Raman effect. Photons can lose part of the energy and are red-shifted or gain energy and are blue-shifted. In biological specimens, photon shifting provides information about conformation, composition and intermolecular interaction in macromolecules (e.g. DNA-protein). There are a few reports on application of this technique to study molecular interactions in individual sperm cells (Huser et al., 2009; Mallidis et al., 2011; Meister et al., 2010). Huser et al. (2009) used Raman spectroscopy to obtain spectra from individual human sperm and reported that there are vibrational marker modes that can be valuable to assess sperm chromatin packaging. Results from this study also indicate that the DNA packaging in sperm with abnormal shape differs from that in normal sperm. In other study (Mallidis et al., 2011), Raman spectra were obtained from individual sperm cells before and after exposition to UVB radiation. Through the analysis of the spectra it was possible to detect the sites and location of UVB-induced sperm DNA damage (Mallidis et al., 2011). Further studies are warranted in order to establish a possible relationship between sperm DNA packaging/damage (as detected by Raman spectrometry) and sperm function at fertilization and beyond.

2.6.5.2 Confocal light absorption and scattering microscopy (CLASS)

Confocal light absorption and scattering microscopy (CLASS) is an optical system that combines confocal microscopy, a well-established high magnification microscopic technique, with light-scattering spectroscopy (Fang et al., 2007). This combination allows for observation of submicrometer structures in viable cells attaining the spatial resolution of electron microscopy without the need of contrasting agents which are required for conventional optical microscopy. Results from studies in biological systems demonstrated that through the use of CLASS technique it is feasible to monitor individual organelles, such as mitochondria, lysosomes and microsomes in living cells (Itzkan et al., 2007). To our knowledge there is no published work regarding the use of CLASS microscopy to study sperm ultrastructure.

2.6.5.3 Sperm chemotaxis

Mammalian spermatozoa have the ability to be actively guided to the egg (that resides at fertilization site) by mechanisms known as chemotaxis and thermotaxis (Eisenbach & Giojalas, 2006). Chemotaxis is the movement of cells following a concentration gradient of chemoattractans whereas thermotaxis is the movement of cells along a temperature gradient. Experimental data support the hypothesis that progesterone (at pM concentrations), secreted by oocyte cumulus cells, is the major chemoattractant for human (Teves et al., 2006) and rabbit spermatozoa (Guidobaldi et al., 2008). Since only a small fraction of capacitated spermatozoa are chemotactically responsive in in vitro assays, it is tempting to hypothesize that the population with enhanced ability to migrate to the chemoattractant source is endowed with superior morphologic/functional features. Based on this principle, a microchannel-based device to assess sperm motility and chemotxis has been recently developed (Xie et al., 2010). However, the impact of using chemotaxis-selected sperm on ART outcomes is currently unknown.

3. Conclusion

Since the world's first "test-tube" baby was born in Great Britain in 1978 (Steptoe & Edwards, 1978), we have witnessed a tremendous progress in the field of human ART which is reflected in the high rates of success accomplished in infertility treatments. Despite these advances, live birth rates achieved by assisted conception remain relatively low and could be improved (Wright et al., 2008). In light of the known influence of the fertilizing spermatozoon not only on early but also on late embryonic development, selection of the best sperm from heterogeneous sperm samples would impact positively on the outcomes of human ARTs. Accurate identification of normal/healthy spermatozoa is of especial importance during ICSI, in which a sperm cell is deliberately injected into the mature oocyte by the technician bypassing all natural barriers. There is great concern about the risk of using sperm with chromosomal abnormalities and/or damaged DNA what can lead to inadvertently transmission of genetic diseases to the offspring. Therefore, improvements of the available sperm selection techniques and/or development of new methods for precise sperm selection are highly desirable. Despite encouraging preliminary results obtained with advanced sperm selection techniques, more research is warranted to address safety issues before widespread application of these methods. In this regard, animal models can provide answers to important safety concerns related to the introduction of advanced and emerging methods for sperm selection into human ART.

4. References

Ainsworth, C., Nixon, B. & Aitken, R. J. (2005). Development of a novel electrophoretic system for the isolation of human spermatozoa. Hum Reprod, Vol.20, No.8, pp. 2261-70, ISSN 0268-1161 (Print) 0268-1161 (Linking)

Ainsworth, C., Nixon, B., Jansen, R. P. & Aitken, R. J. (2007). First recorded pregnancy and normal birth after ICSI using electrophoretically isolated spermatozoa. Hum Reprod, Vol.22, No.1, pp. 197-200, ISSN 0268-1161 (Print) 0268-1161 (Linking)

Ainsworth, C. J., Nixon, B. & Aitken, R. J. (2011). The electrophoretic separation of spermatozoa: an analysis of genotype, surface carbohydrate composition and potential for capacitation. Int J Androl, Vol.34, No.5 Pt 2, pp. e422-34, ISSN 1365-2605 (Electronic) 0105-6263 (Linking)

Angelopoulos, T., Moshel, Y. A., Lu, L., Macanas, E., Grifo, J. A. & Krey, L. C. (1998). Simultaneous assessment of sperm chromatin condensation and morphology before and after separation procedures: effect on the clinical outcome after in vitro fertilization. Fertil Steril, Vol.69, No.4, pp. 740-7, ISSN 0015-0282 (Print) 0015-0282 (Linking)

Avendano, C., Franchi, A., Duran, H. & Oehninger, S. (2010). DNA fragmentation of normal spermatozoa negatively impacts embryo quality and intracytoplasmic sperm injection outcome. Fertil Steril, Vol.94, No.2, pp. 549-57, ISSN 1556-5653 (Electronic) 0015-0282 (Linking)

Avendano, C., Franchi, A., Taylor, S., Morshedi, M., Bocca, S. & Oehninger, S. (2009). Fragmentation of DNA in morphologically normal human spermatozoa. Fertil Steril, Vol.91, No.4, pp. 1077-84, ISSN 1556-5653 (Electronic) 0015-0282 (Linking)

Avendano, C. & Oehninger, S. (2011). DNA fragmentation in morphologically normal spermatozoa: how much should we be concerned in the ICSI era? J Androl, Vol.32, No.4, pp. 356-63, ISSN 1939-4640 (Electronic) 0196-3635 (Linking)

Baccetti, B. (2004). Microscopical advances in assisted reproduction. J Submicrosc Cytol Pathol, Vol.36, No.3-4, pp. 333-9, ISSN 1122-9497 (Print) 1122-9497 (Linking)

Barroso, G., Valdespin, C., Vega, E., Kershenovich, R., Avila, R., Avendano, C. & Oehninger, S. (2009). Developmental sperm contributions: fertilization and beyond. Fertil Steril, Vol.92, No.3, pp. 835-48, ISSN 1556-5653 (Electronic) 0015-0282 (Linking)

Bartoov, B., Berkovitz, A., Eltes, F., Kogosovsky, A., Yagoda, A., Lederman, H., Artzi, S., Gross, M. & Barak, Y. (2003). Pregnancy rates are higher with intracytoplasmic morphologically selected sperm injection than with conventional intracytoplasmic injection. Fertil Steril, Vol.80, No.6, pp. 1413-9, ISSN 0015-0282 (Print) 0015-0282 (Linking)

Bartoov, B., Berkovitz, A., Eltes, F., Kogosowski, A., Menezo, Y. & Barak, Y. (2002). Real-time fine morphology of motile human sperm cells is associated with IVF-ICSI outcome. J Androl, Vol.23, No.1, pp. 1-8, ISSN 0196-3635 (Print) 0196-3635 (Linking)

Bjorndahl, L., Mohammadieh, M., Pourian, M., Soderlund, I. & Kvist, U. (2005). Contamination by seminal plasma factors during sperm selection. J Androl, Vol.26, No.2, pp. 170-3, ISSN 0196-3635 (Print) 0196-3635 (Linking)

Chan, P. J., Jacobson, J. D., Corselli, J. U. & Patton, W. C. (2006). A simple zeta method for sperm selection based on membrane charge. Fertil Steril, Vol.85, No.2, pp. 481-6, ISSN 1556-5653 (Electronic) 0015-0282 (Linking)

Dirican, E. K., Ozgun, O. D., Akarsu, S., Akin, K. O., Ercan, O., Ugurlu, M., Camsari, C., Kanyilmaz, O., Kaya, A. & Unsal, A. (2008). Clinical outcome of magnetic activated cell sorting of non-apoptotic spermatozoa before density gradient centrifugation for assisted reproduction. J Assist Reprod Genet, Vol.25, No.8, pp. 375-81, ISSN 1058-0468 (Print) 1058-0468 (Linking)

Edwards, R. G., Bavister, B. D. & Steptoe, P. C. (1969). Early stages of fertilization in vitro of human oocytes matured in vitro. Nature, Vol.221, No.5181, pp. 632-5, ISSN 0028-0836 (Print) 0028-0836 (Linking)

Eisenbach, M. & Giojalas, L. C. (2006). Sperm guidance in mammals - an unpaved road to the egg. Nat Rev Mol Cell Biol, Vol.7, No.4, pp. 276-85, ISSN 1471-0072 (Print) 1471-0072 (Linking)

Fang, H., Qiu, L., Vitkin, E., Zaman, M. M., Andersson, C., Salahuddin, S., Kimerer, L. M., Cipolloni, P. B., Modell, M. D., Turner, B. S., Keates, S. E., Bigio, I., Itzkan, I., Freedman, S. D., Bansil, R., Hanlon, E. B. & Perelman, L. T. (2007). Confocal light absorption and scattering spectroscopic microscopy. Appl Opt, Vol.46, No.10, pp. 1760-9, ISSN 0003-6935 (Print) 0003-6935 (Linking)

Fleming, S. D., Ilad, R. S., Griffin, A. M., Wu, Y., Ong, K. J., Smith, H. C. & Aitken, R. J. (2008). Prospective controlled trial of an electrophoretic method of sperm preparation for assisted reproduction: comparison with density gradient centrifugation. Hum Reprod, Vol.23, No.12, pp. 2646-51, ISSN 1460-2350 (Electronic) 0268-1161 (Linking)

Ford, W. (1990). The role of oxygen free radicals in the pathology of human spermatozoa: Implications of IVF. In Clinical IVF Forum; Current Views in Assisted Reproduction, (ed. P. Matson & B. Lieberman), pp. 123-139: Manchester University Press.

Gianaroli, L., Magli, M. C., Collodel, G., Moretti, E., Ferraretti, A. P. & Baccetti, B. (2008). Sperm head's birefringence: a new criterion for sperm selection. Fertil Steril, Vol.90, No.1, pp. 104-12, ISSN 1556-5653 (Electronic) 0015-0282 (Linking)

Gianaroli, L., Magli, M. C., Ferraretti, A. P., Crippa, A., Lappi, M., Capitani, S. & Baccetti, B. (2010). Birefringence characteristics in sperm heads allow for the selection of reacted spermatozoa for intracytoplasmic sperm injection. Fertil Steril, Vol.93, No.3, pp. 807-13, ISSN 1556-5653 (Electronic) 0015-0282 (Linking)

Giuliani, V., Pandolfi, C., Santucci, R., Pelliccione, F., Macerola, B., Focarelli, R., Rosati, F., Della Giovampaola, C., Francavilla, F. & Francavilla, S. (2004). Expression of gp20, a human sperm antigen of epididymal origin, is reduced in spermatozoa from subfertile men. Mol Reprod Dev, Vol.69, No.2, pp. 235-40, ISSN 1040-452X (Print) 1040-452X (Linking)

Grunewald, S., Paasch, U. & Glander, H. J. (2001). Enrichment of non-apoptotic human spermatozoa after cryopreservation by immunomagnetic cell sorting. Cell Tissue Bank, Vol.2, No.3, pp. 127-33, ISSN 1573-6814 (Electronic) 1389-9333 (Linking)

Guidobaldi, H. A., Teves, M. E., Unates, D. R., Anastasia, A. & Giojalas, L. C. (2008). Progesterone from the cumulus cells is the sperm chemoattractant secreted by the rabbit oocyte cumulus complex. PLoS One, Vol.3, No.8, pp. e3040, ISSN 1932-6203 (Electronic) 1932-6203 (Linking)

Hallap, T., Haard, M., Jaakma, U., Larsson, B. & Rodriguez-Martinez, H. (2004). Does cleansing of frozen-thawed bull semen before assessment provide samples that relate better to potential fertility? Theriogenology, Vol.62, No.3-4, pp. 702-13, ISSN 0093-691X (Print) 0093-691X (Linking)

Henkel, R., Kierspel, E., Stalf, T., Mehnert, C., Menkveld, R., Tinneberg, H. R., Schill, W. B. & Kruger, T. F. (2005). Effect of reactive oxygen species produced by spermatozoa and leukocytes on sperm functions in non-leukocytospermic patients. Fertil Steril, Vol.83, No.3, pp. 635-42, ISSN 0015-0282 (Print) 0015-0282 (Linking)

Henkel, R. R. & Schill, W. B. (2003). Sperm preparation for ART. Reprod Biol Endocrinol, Vol.1, pp. 108, ISSN 1477-7827 (Electronic) 1477-7827 (Linking)

Hinting, A. & Lunardhi, H. (2001). Better sperm selection for intracytoplasmic sperm injection with the side migration technique. Andrologia, Vol.33, No.6, pp. 343-6, ISSN 0303-4569 (Print) 0303-4569 (Linking)

Huser, T., Orme, C. A., Hollars, C. W., Corzett, M. H. & Balhorn, R. (2009). Raman spectroscopy of DNA packaging in individual human sperm cells distinguishes normal from abnormal cells. J Biophotonics, Vol.2, No.5, pp. 322-32, ISSN 1864-0648 (Electronic) 1864-063X (Linking)

Huszar, G., Jakab, A., Sakkas, D., Ozenci, C. C., Cayli, S., Delpiano, E. & Ozkavukcu, S. (2007). Fertility testing and ICSI sperm selection by hyaluronic acid binding: clinical and genetic aspects. Reprod Biomed Online, Vol.14, No.5, pp. 650-63, ISSN 1472-6483 (Print) 1472-6483 (Linking)

Huszar, G., Ozenci, C. C., Cayli, S., Zavaczki, Z., Hansch, E. & Vigue, L. (2003). Hyaluronic acid binding by human sperm indicates cellular maturity, viability, and unreacted acrosomal status. Fertil Steril, Vol.79 Suppl 3, pp. 1616-24, ISSN 0015-0282 (Print) 0015-0282 (Linking)

Ishijima, S. A., Okuno, M. & Mohri, H. (1991). Zeta potential of human X- and Y-bearing sperm. Int J Androl, Vol.14, No.5, pp. 340-7, ISSN 0105-6263 (Print) 0105-6263 (Linking)

Itzkan, I., Qiu, L., Fang, H., Zaman, M. M., Vitkin, E., Ghiran, I. C., Salahuddin, S., Modell, M., Andersson, C., Kimerer, L. M., Cipolloni, P. B., Lim, K. H., Freedman, S. D., Bigio, I., Sachs, B. P., Hanlon, E. B. & Perelman, L. T. (2007). Confocal light absorption and scattering spectroscopic microscopy monitors organelles in live cells with no exogenous labels. Proc Natl Acad Sci U S A, Vol.104, No.44, pp. 17255-60, ISSN 0027-8424 (Print) 0027-8424 (Linking)

Jakab, A., Sakkas, D., Delpiano, E., Cayli, S., Kovanci, E., Ward, D., Revelli, A. & Huszar, G. (2005). Intracytoplasmic sperm injection: a novel selection method for sperm with normal frequency of chromosomal aneuploidies. Fertil Steril, Vol.84, No.6, pp. 1665-73, ISSN 1556-5653 (Electronic) 0015-0282 (Linking)

Kheirollahi-Kouhestani, M., Razavi, S., Tavalaee, M., Deemeh, M. R., Mardani, M., Moshtaghian, J. & Nasr-Esfahani, M. H. (2009). Selection of sperm based on combined density gradient and Zeta method may improve ICSI outcome. Hum Reprod, Vol.24, No.10, pp. 2409-16, ISSN 1460-2350 (Electronic) 0268-1161 (Linking)

Lee, T. H., Liu, C. H., Shih, Y. T., Tsao, H. M., Huang, C. C., Chen, H. H. & Lee, M. S. (2010). Magnetic-activated cell sorting for sperm preparation reduces spermatozoa with apoptotic markers and improves the acrosome reaction in couples with unexplained infertility. Hum Reprod, Vol.25, No.4, pp. 839-46, ISSN 1460-2350 (Electronic) 0268-1161 (Linking)

Lopata, A., Brown, J. B., Leeton, J. F., Talbot, J. M. & Wood, C. (1978). In vitro fertilization of preovulatory oocytes and embryo transfer in infertile patients treated with clomiphene and human chorionic gonadotropin. Fertil Steril, Vol.30, No.1, pp. 27-35, ISSN 0015-0282 (Print) 0015-0282 (Linking)

Mahadevan, M. & Baker, G. (1984). Assessment and preparation of semen for in vitro fertilization. In Clinical In Vitro Fertilization, (ed. C. Wood & A. Trounson), pp. 83-97. Berlin: Springer-Verlag.

Mallidis, C., Wistuba, J., Bleisteiner, B., Damm, O. S., Gross, P., Wubbeling, F., Fallnich, C., Burger, M. & Schlatt, S. (2011). In situ visualization of damaged DNA in human sperm by Raman microspectroscopy. Hum Reprod, Vol.26, No.7, pp. 1641-9, ISSN 1460-2350 (Electronic) 0268-1161 (Linking)

Manz, R., Assenmacher, M., Pfluger, E., Miltenyi, S. & Radbruch, A. (1995). Analysis and sorting of live cells according to secreted molecules, relocated to a cell-surface affinity matrix. Proc Natl Acad Sci U S A, Vol.92, No.6, pp. 1921-5, ISSN 0027-8424 (Print) 0027-8424 (Linking)

Meister, K., Schmidt, D. A., Brundermann, E. & Havenith, M. (2010). Confocal Raman microspectroscopy as an analytical tool to assess the mitochondrial status in human spermatozoa. Analyst, Vol.135, No.6, pp. 1370-4, ISSN 1364-5528 (Electronic) 0003-2654 (Linking)

Moohan, J. M. & Lindsay, K. S. (1995). Spermatozoa selected by a discontinuous Percoll density gradient exhibit better motion characteristics, more hyperactivation, and longer survival than direct swim-up. Fertil Steril, Vol.64, No.1, pp. 160-5, ISSN 0015-0282 (Print) 0015-0282 (Linking)

Morrell, J. M., Garcia, B. M., Pena, F. J. & Johannisson, A. (2011). Processing stored stallion semen doses by Single Layer Centrifugation. Theriogenology, Vol.76, No.8, pp. 1424-32, ISSN 1879-3231 (Electronic) 0093-691X (Linking)

Mortimer, D. (2000). Sperm preparation methods. J Androl, Vol.21, No.3, pp. 357-66, ISSN 0196-3635 (Print) 0196-3635 (Linking)

Nasr-Esfahani, M. H., Razavi, S., Vahdati, A. A., Fathi, F. & Tavalaee, M. (2008). Evaluation of sperm selection procedure based on hyaluronic acid binding ability on ICSI outcome. J Assist Reprod Genet, Vol.25, No.5, pp. 197-203, ISSN 1058-0468 (Print) 1058-0468 (Linking)

Parmegiani, L., Cognigni, G. E., Bernardi, S., Troilo, E., Ciampaglia, W. & Filicori, M. (2010a). "Physiologic ICSI": hyaluronic acid (HA) favors selection of spermatozoa without DNA fragmentation and with normal nucleus, resulting in improvement of embryo quality. Fertil Steril, Vol.93, No.2, pp. 598-604, ISSN 1556-5653 (Electronic) 0015-0282 (Linking)

Parmegiani, L., Cognigni, G. E., Ciampaglia, W., Pocognoli, P., Marchi, F. & Filicori, M. (2010b). Efficiency of hyaluronic acid (HA) sperm selection. J Assist Reprod Genet, Vol.27, No.1, pp. 13-6, ISSN 1573-7330 (Electronic) 1058-0468 (Linking)

Said, T., Agarwal, A., Grunewald, S., Rasch, M., Baumann, T., Kriegel, C., Li, L., Glander, H. J., Thomas, A. J., Jr. & Paasch, U. (2006a). Selection of nonapoptotic spermatozoa as a new tool for enhancing assisted reproduction outcomes: an in vitro model. Biol Reprod, Vol.74, No.3, pp. 530-7, ISSN 0006-3363 (Print) 0006-3363 (Linking)

Said, T. M., Agarwal, A., Grunewald, S., Rasch, M., Glander, H. J. & Paasch, U. (2006b). Evaluation of sperm recovery following annexin V magnetic-activated cell sorting separation. Reprod Biomed Online, Vol.13, No.3, pp. 336-9, ISSN 1472-6483 (Print) 1472-6483 (Linking)

Said, T. M., Agarwal, A., Zborowski, M., Grunewald, S., Glander, H. J. & Paasch, U. (2008). Utility of magnetic cell separation as a molecular sperm preparation technique. J Androl, Vol.29, No.2, pp. 134-42, ISSN 0196-3635 (Print) 0196-3635 (Linking)

Said, T. M., Grunewald, S., Paasch, U., Glander, H. J., Baumann, T., Kriegel, C., Li, L. & Agarwal, A. (2005a). Advantage of combining magnetic cell separation with sperm preparation techniques. Reprod Biomed Online, Vol.10, No.6, pp. 740-6, ISSN 1472-6483 (Print) 1472-6483 (Linking)

Said, T. M., Grunewald, S., Paasch, U., Rasch, M., Agarwal, A. & Glander, H. J. (2005b). Effects of magnetic-activated cell sorting on sperm motility and cryosurvival rates. Fertil Steril, Vol.83, No.5, pp. 1442-6, ISSN 1556-5653 (Electronic) 0015-0282 (Linking)

Sakkas, D., Manicardi, G. C., Tomlinson, M., Mandrioli, M., Bizzaro, D., Bianchi, P. G. & Bianchi, U. (2000). The use of two density gradient centrifugation techniques and the swim-up method to separate spermatozoa with chromatin and nuclear DNA anomalies. Hum Reprod, Vol.15, No.5, pp. 1112-6, ISSN 0268-1161 (Print) 0268-1161 (Linking)

Schroter, S., Derr, P., Conradt, H. S., Nimtz, M., Hale, G. & Kirchhoff, C. (1999). Male-specific modification of human CD52. J Biol Chem, Vol.274, No.42, pp. 29862-73, ISSN 0021-9258 (Print) 0021-9258 (Linking)

Souza Setti, A., Ferreira, R. C., Paes de Almeida Ferreira Braga, D., de Cassia Savio Figueira, R., Iaconelli, A., Jr. & Borges, E., Jr. (2010). Intracytoplasmic sperm injection outcome versus intracytoplasmic morphologically selected sperm injection outcome: a meta-analysis. Reprod Biomed Online, Vol.21, No.4, pp. 450-5, ISSN 1472-6491 (Electronic) 1472-6483 (Linking)

Steptoe, P. C. & Edwards, R. G. (1978). Birth after the reimplantation of a human embryo. Lancet, Vol.2, No.8085, pp. 366, ISSN 0140-6736 (Print) 0140-6736 (Linking)

Tea, N., Jondet, M. & Scholler, R. (1984). A migration-gravity sedimentation method for collecting motile spermatozoa from human semen. In: In Vitro Fertilization, Embryo Transfer and Early Pregnancy, R. Harrison J. Bonnar & W. Thompson (Ed.), MTP Press ltd, Lancaster

Teves, M. E., Barbano, F., Guidobaldi, H. A., Sanchez, R., Miska, W. & Giojalas, L. C. (2006). Progesterone at the picomolar range is a chemoattractant for mammalian spermatozoa. Fertil Steril, Vol.86, No.3, pp. 745-9, ISSN 1556-5653 (Electronic) 0015-0282 (Linking)

Tomlinson, M. J., Moffatt, O., Manicardi, G. C., Bizzaro, D., Afnan, M. & Sakkas, D. (2001). Interrelationships between seminal parameters and sperm nuclear DNA damage before and after density gradient centrifugation: implications for assisted conception. Hum Reprod, Vol.16, No.10, pp. 2160-5, ISSN 0268-1161 (Print) 0268-1161 (Linking)

Wikland, M., Wik, O., Steen, Y., Qvist, K., Soderlund, B. & Janson, P. O. (1987). A self-migration method for preparation of sperm for in-vitro fertilization. Hum Reprod, Vol.2, No.3, pp. 191-5, ISSN 0268-1161 (Print) 0268-1161 (Linking)

Wright, V. C., Chang, J., Jeng, G. & Macaluso, M. (2008). Assisted reproductive technology surveillance--United States, 2005. MMWR Surveill Summ, Vol.57, No.5, pp. 1-23, ISSN 1545-8636 (Electronic) 0892-3787 (Linking)

Xie, L., Ma, R., Han, C., Su, K., Zhang, Q., Qiu, T., Wang, L., Huang, G., Qiao, J., Wang, J. & Cheng, J. (2010). Integration of sperm motility and chemotaxis screening with a microchannel-based device. Clin Chem, Vol.56, No.8, pp. 1270-8, ISSN 1530-8561 (Electronic) 0009-9147 (Linking)

5

Analysis of Permissive and Repressive Chromatin Markers in *In Vitro* Fertilized Bovine Embryos Just After Embryonic Genome Activation

Clara Slade Oliveira, Naiara Zoccal Saraiva,
Letícia Zoccolaro Oliveira and Joaquim Mansano Garcia
São Paulo State University (UNESP Jaboticabal)
Brazil

1. Introduction

Preimplantation development in mammalian species is a challenging stage of embryogenesis, which makes in vitro fertilization and embryo culture sophisticated biotechniques. One of the main tasks is to provide cultured embryos an adequate environment that allows embryonic-maternal transition, and consequent achievement of an independent gene expression program.

In this respect, mammalian models have been used to further elucidate the mechanisms of embryonic genome activation. Within the main players in this context we can include chromatin compactor/relaxing agents, and among them histone modifying enzymes and their consequent posttranslational modifications.

In this chapter, we aim to discuss some histone modification marks observed during embryonic genome activation, and how their monitoring can provide useful information about early embryo development.

1.1 In Vitro Production (IVP) of mammalian embryos: How other species can contribute to human IVP improvement

In vitro early embryo development was first established in human species in 1978 and represented an important achievement for Reproductive Medicine. However, despite several decades of research and clinical experience, in vitro development of blastocysts and pregnancy following embryo transfer has not been yet fully dominated. Although improvements of medium, atmosphere, hormone stimulation, oocyte recovery and embryo transfer protocols were achieved during the last 30 years, rates of in vitro developed blastocysts are still around 40% in most systems (Bannister & Kouzarides, 2011; Bolton et al., 1991; Hardy et al., 1989; Zhang et al., 2010). Furthermore, the identification of developmentally competent embryos is still a difficult task.

Among several critical steps of IVP, one that has the most stochastic consequence is the activation of embryonic genome. At this time point, a phenomenon observed in many species is the developmental block of embryos due to the inability to activate zygotic genes and continue cleavage. As the usage of human embryos for research involves major ethical issues, most researches are conducted in other mammalian models. In this context, despite several advantages of mouse physiology as a model for human development, bovine early embryo development presents more similarities to human at some aspects.

Mouse embryos develop to the blastocyst stage in 3.5 days and the rate of blastocyst production in most labs is about 90%. Furthermore, developmental block during embryonic genome activation (EGA) is not a common phenomenon for most mouse embryos, occurring normally to only some inbreed mice strains (Shire & Whitten, 1980). On the contrary, one of the main causes of embryonic arrest for bovine embryos appears to be the inability to overcome chromatin repression before maternal RNAs stock has been depleted, which occurs approximately by the 8cell stage (Meirelles et al., 2004). Failure to activate zygotic genome on time is also an issue for human embryos, and most arresting embryos stop development at this time point (Artley et al., 1992). The timing of EGA is also closer between bovine (8-16cell) (Badr et al., 2007) and human (4-8 cell) (Braude et al., 1988) embryos, which corresponds to day 3 of embryonic development in both bovine (Oliveira et al., 2010) and human (Sepulveda et al., 2011) embryos.

The reason why embryonic block does not affect most of mouse embryos might be related to the fact that EGA initiates in this species just a few hours after fertilization (Hamatani et al., 2004), while for bovine and human embryos it takes up to 3 days. In fact, the lower rates of blastocysts observed for bovine and human comparing to mouse embryos might be as well a result of extended IVC, since culture environment can affect epigenetic modifications pattern (Enright et al., 2003). This aspect may contribute to the different gene transcription profiles observed between bovine embryos produced in vitro and in vivo (Wrenzycki et al., 2004). In IVF embryos, some genes are expressed at a low level, such as transcripts associated with compactation/cavitation (Wrenzycki et al., 1996), stress adaptation (Rizos et al., 2002), embryonic metabolism (Bertolini et al., 2002), and X chromosome inactivation (Wrenzycki et al., 2002).

Therefore, bovine embryogenesis seems to be an appropriate model for studying histone modifications in human pre implantation development, including in vitro embryonic genome activation. We believe that epigenetic marks can reflect developmental competence, and also that the manipulation of those epigenetic states might be useful to elucidate their roles during mammalian early embryo development.

1.2 Maternal-zygotic transition: Achievement of an independent gene expression program

1.2.1 Degradation of maternal mRNAs transcripts

The oocyte is the largest mammalian cell, and has an extensive amount of cytoplasm comprising an abundant reserve of RNAs. After oocyte maturation, nuclei is arrested in metaphase, when transcription stops and translation is reduced. The huge amount of RNA accumulated during oocyte growth is then kept and utilized during the first embryonic divisions as a maternal stock (Lonergan et al., 2003). Those maternal RNAs are essential for embryonic development until the event of EGA occurs, as they provide most translational elements used for protein synthesis during initial divisions. Therefore, adequate availability of maternal transcripts should be present until that moment, which also explain why oocyte quality is so important for species which EGA occurs 2 or more cell cycles after fertilization, as in bovine embryos (Meirelles et al., 2004).

The first few days of oocyte maturation and embryo development in human are characterized by a significant decrease in transcript levels, including pro apoptotic genes, suggesting that decay of those maternal RNAs are essential for embryo development (Dobson et al., 2004). Such a staged down regulation has not been reported for any organism during early development, and it is not clear whether it is required for genome activation to occur, or whether it is an independent event in early embryo development. Vassena et al. (2011) reported this maternal mRNA turnover to occur in two waves, tiled during early development. The first wave, termed 'early maternal', probably takes place between the Metaphase II (MII) and 2-cell stage, and during this time, maternal mRNAs are loaded onto polysomes, translocated and degraded. A second wave of maternal mRNA degradation, termed 'late maternal', included transcripts that decrease gradually over time.

1.2.2 Activation of embryonic genome

Embryonic genome activation timing differs between mammalian species. It occurs at the 2-cell stage in mouse (Bensaude et al., 1983; Moore, 1975), at the 4- to 8-cell stage in horse (Brinsko et al., 1995) and human (Braude et al., 1988), and at the 8- to 16-cell stage in cow (De Sousa et al., 1998), sheep (Crosby et al., 1988), rabbit (Brunet-Simon et al., 2001) and monkey (Schramm & Bavister, 1999). Maternal-zygotic transition is essential for the activation of a large number of genes, thus achieving a gene expression pattern compatible with embryonic development and differentiation (Schultz, 2002).

Most studies involving EGA are carried out in mouse embryos. In this species, the first signs of zygotic transcriptional activity occur few hours after fertilization, before first cleavage, mainly in the male pronucleus (Aoki et al., 1997; Nothias et al., 1996). This wave is named Minor Zygotic Activation (Minor ZGA), and it is responsible for a small set of peptides that are transiently increased by the 2cell stage. Then, during transition from 2 to 4 cell stage, a dramatic increase in transcriptional activity is described, entitled Major Zygotic Activation (Major ZGA), and embryonic gene expression pattern is established. Embryos that fail to activate their own genome are arrested (Rambhatla & Latham, 1995). At this moment, genes that encode basic cellular machinery are activated (Davis & Schultz, 1997). Nonetheless, embryonic genome must suffer a third wave of transcription activation at the 4cell stage. This wave represents the second major transition of gene expression profile, and is named mid pre-implantational gene activation (Hamatani et al., 2006). At this point, genes associated with critical function in early embryos, such as key regulators for epiblast (EPI) and trophectoderm (TE) specification, are activated.

Human EGA was first described during the transition from 4- to 8- cell stages (Tesarík et al., 1988). However, Vassena et al. (2011) recently identified transcriptional activity in the human embryo at the 2-cell stage. The authors also identified three waves of transcriptional activation in the human embryo: at 2-cell stage, 4-cell stage, and between the 6- and the 8- to 10-cell stages. The major wave, which the authors interpreted as similar to Major ZGA in mouse, occurred between the 8-10 cell stages. In bovine, Minor ZGA is described from 1- to

4-cell stage, but major transition, which is responsible for embryonic developmental competence, occurs during the transition from the 8-16cell stage (Badr et al., 2007).

In conclusion, we can observe that embryonic genome activity is dramatically transformed in just a few days, or even hours. Those transcriptional profiles reflect chromatin architecture and compaction, which is built in part by chromatin modifications. In the next topic, we will address how histone modifications can play a role in embryonic genome activation.

1.3 Epigenetic mechanisms during early embryo development

Epigenetic refers to the control of gene function and expression without changing genomic sequence. This regulation allows the existence of tissue-specific gene expression patterns within one organism (Li, 2002). Epigenetic modifications can control gene expression by a range of processes which include DNA methylation, post-translational histone modifications and non-coding RNAs. Covalent modifications of histones occurs on amino residues, primarily on the amino-terminal tail (Bannister & Kouzarides, 2011), and have fundamental functions on chromatin condensation, DNA replication, DNA repair, and gene regulation. Therefore, based on biochemical interaction, histone modifications can induce chromatin decondensation, allowing transcription factors to bind, or maintain nucleosomes tightly wound.

Examples of some modifications that are commonly associated with active sites of transcription are acetylation of histone H3 and H4, as well as di- and trimethylation of lysine 4 on histone H3 (Kouzarides, 2007). On the other hand, constitutively silenced DNA regions such as telomere, centromeres, and heterochromatin are hypoacetylated and highly methylated on particular amino acid residues (lysine 9 and lysine 27 of histone H3).

Among histone modifications, acetylation and methylation have been so far the most described. Unlike histone acetylation, that is always associated with transcriptional activation, histone methylation can induce different outcomes depending on which residue is modified (Martin & Zhang, 2005). Both modifications are conducted by enzymes. For acetylation, histone acetyltransferase (HAT; adds acetyl groups) and histone deacetylase (HDAC; removes acetyls groups) are involved on lysine regulation (Wolffe & Guschin, 2000). Several of these enzymes (HDACs 1, 2, 3, 7, and HAT1) have been detected in bovine embryos (McGraw et al., 2003), and as more research is conducted, it becomes apparent that crosstalk between enzymes is a common feature.

Therefore, a wide array of epigenetic modifications participates in early embryo development, including DNA methylation and histone modifications, and they are crucial for genomic imprinting and X-chromosome inactivation in female embryos (Dean et al., 2003). Time course studies demonstrate that those modifications are switched between embryonic stages and are well orchestrated to warrant normal development. For instance, levels of histone methylation are higher and histone acetylation levels are lower in male gametes compared to female gametes (Adenot et al., 1997; Kim et al., 2003; Sarmento et al., 2004; Spinaci et al., 2004), resulting in minimal gene expression at this stage. Then, demethylation occurs soon after fertilization (Sanz et al., 2010). Histone methylation levels are reduced in 2 to 4 cell embryos, and start to increase at the 8- to 16-cell stage, concurrently with zygotic genome activation (Santos et al., 2003). Histone acetylation levels peak at the time of zygotic genome activation, corresponding to a dramatic increase in gene expression levels, and then diminishes during the morula stage (Maalouf et al., 2008).

At the blastocyst stage, DNA and histone methylation are elevated in the ICM, whereas DNA and histones are hypomethylated in the trophectoderm, which clearly reflects a difference between the two cell lineages (Reik et al., 2003). However, studies suggest that this epigenetic status segregation can occur even before. It has been demonstrated that chromatin modifications are differentially distributed between blastomeres as early as at 4-cell stage. Torres-Padilla et al. (2007) described CARM1 enzyme, a histone H3 arginine methyltransferase, as being involved in pluripotency achievement. Furthermore, methylation of arginine histone H3 residues is increased in 4-cell blastomeres that will contribute to ICM formation. Thus, histone modifications are involved in lineage specification in early embryos, and seems to occur earlier than most events related to embryo differentiation.

In addition, studies have demonstrated that histone modifications are disrupted by embryo manipulation and in vitro culture. Santos et al. (2003) demonstrated that bovine embryos produced by somatic cell nuclear transfer (SCNT) presented hypermethylation of histone H3-K9. A study also reported that acetylation of lysine 5 on histone H4 (H4-K5ac) appears to change dramatically during early embryo development of IVF produced embryos, but remains consistently elevated in SCNT produced bovine embryos (Kang et al., 2002).

Compared to in vitro fertilized embryos, SCNT bovine embryos have elevated heterochromatic histone methylation (H3K9me2) and H3K9-acetylation in the trophoectoderm layer (Santos et al., 2003). These and other modifications could explain the altered expression of vital developmental genes later in development. Bovine cultured cells also present a disrupted pattern of epigenetic modifications (Enright et al., 2003). In this respect, we described that it is possible to artificially increase histone acetylation during in vitro culture. Trichostatin A (TSA), a histone deacetylase inhibitor, can be added to culture medium at low concentrations without causing detrimental effects to embryonic development (Oliveira et al., 2011).

Embryos cultured in TSA supplemented medium present higher acetylation levels, and develop normally. Furthermore, female and male embryos respond to TSA treatment in a different way (Oliveira et al., 2010), and this might be related to X chromosome inactivation event (unpublished results).

In conclusion, epigenetic modifications are essential during early embryo development, and they have a predictable and well orchestrated pattern of expression which correlates with developmental potencial, and seems to influence lineage specification. It has been demonstrated that manipulation of embryos leads to disruption in histone modifications pattern, as we summarized in this topic. Therefore, monitoring of histone post-translational modifications during preimplantation development is an important tool for assessing culture environment. In addition, a better understanding of how those modifications can be manipulated might be even more interesting aiming the achievement of improved phenotype blastocysts and ES cells derivation, in terms of pluripotent capacity of inner cell mass. In this respect, we are studying concomitantly two well described histone modifications, H3k9ac (permissive chromatin) and H3k27me3 (repressive chromatin), in bovine embryos. At this stage, we aimed to describe how they correlate and are distributed during EGA, comparing blastomeres within one embryo.

2. In Vitro Production (IVP) of bovine embryos

Development of bovine embryos in vitro for research purposes is mainly carried out using oocytes obtained from slaughterhouse ovaries. Blastocyst production includes oocyte maturation, in vitro fertilization and embryo culture, and can be accomplished in 7-8 days, with rates of approximately 40%. Here we briefly describe all steps of this process.

2.1 Supplements

Reagents and culture media were purchased from Sigma Chemical Co. (St. Louis, MO) unless otherwise stated.

2.2 Preparation and selection of oocytes

Bovine ovaries were collected at a local slaughterhouse and processed within 2 h after slaughter. The ovaries were washed in saline (37°C) and follicles measuring 3 to 8 mm in diameter were aspirated with an 18-gauge needle coupled to a 20-mL syringe. Follicle liquid was placed in a 50 mL conic tube for 20 min sedimentation at 37°C, and then 10 mL of the sediment was collected and transferred to 100 mm Petri dishes. Cumulus-oocyte complexes (COCs) presenting at least three layers of cumulus cells and homogenous cytoplasm were selected under a stereomicroscope. The COCs were washed in HEPES-buffered TCM-199 (Gibco BRL, Grand Island, NY, USA) supplemented with 10% fetal calf serum (FCS; Cripion Biotecnologia, Andradina, SP, Brazil), 16 µg/mL sodium pyruvate and 83.4 µg/mL amikacin (Instituto Biochimico, Rio de Janeiro, RJ, Brazil).

2.3 In vitro maturation (IVM)

Groups of 15 COCs were transferred to 100-µL drops of medium containing sodium bicarbonate-buffered TCM-199 supplemented with 10% FCS, 1.0 µg/mL FSH (Folltropin™, Bioniche Animal Health, Belleville, ON, Canada), 50 µg/mL hCG (Profasi™, Serono, Sao Paulo, SP, Brazil), 1.0 µg/mL estradiol, 16 µg/mL sodium pyruvate and 83.4 µg/mL amikacin, covered with sterile mineral oil (Dow Corning Co., Midland, MI, USA) and incubated for 24 h at 38.5°C in an atmosphere of 5% CO_2 in air under saturated humidity.

2.4 In vitro fertilization (IVF)

After in vitro maturation (IVM) the cumulus cells were partially removed from the oocytes by vigorous pipetting. Groups of 20 oocytes were washed twice and transferred to 80-µL drops of TALP-IVF medium supplemented with 0.6% BSA, 10 µg/mL heparin, 18 µM penicillamine, 10 µM hypotaurine and 1.8 µM epinephrine, and covered with sterile mineral oil. A frozen straw of semen was thawed at 35.5°C and centrifuged on a discontinuous 45/90 Percoll gradient for 7 min at 3600 x *g*. The pellet was collected (100 µL) and resuspended in 700 µL TALP-IVF medium and again centrifuged for 5 min at 520 x *g*. After centrifugation, 30 µL of the medium containing the pellet was collected from the bottom of the tube and homogenized in a conical tube. The suspension was adjusted for a final concentration of approximately 104 mobile spermatozoa for each oocyte. The plates were incubated at 38.5°C for 20 h in an atmosphere of 5% CO_2 in air under saturated humidity. Semen from the same bull and the same batch was used for all replicates.

2.5 In vitro culture (IVC)

After IVF, presumptive zygotes were denuded of cumulus cells by vigorous pipetting. Embryos were washed three times and transferred in groups of 15 to 20 to be cultured in 100-µL drops of SOF medium supplemented with 5 mg/mL BSA and 2.5% FCS. The dishes were then incubated in an atmosphere of 5% O_2 in air under saturated humidity for 5 days at 38° C. The cleavage rate, blastocyst development, and blastocyst hatching were evaluated 48 h, 7 days and 9 days after IVF, respectively.

2.6 Immunocytochemistry of H3K9ac and H3k27me3

For this experiment, we used day 5 embryos, 70h after IVF. At this timepoint, approximately 30-50% of embryos should be at the 5th cell cycle. Embryos were fixed in 4% paraformaldehyde for 30 min at 37°C and stored at 4°C in PBS supplemented with 3% BSA and 0.5% Triton X-100 for up to 1 week. Fixed embryos were incubated in blocking solution (3% BSA and 0.2% Tween-20 in PBS) for 1 h at room temperature. Next, the embryos were incubated with the primary antibodies (mouse anti-H3K9ac monoclonal antibody, 1:200, and rabbit anti-H3k27me3 monoclonal antibody (1:200; Upstate Biotechnology, Lake Placid, NY, USA) for 12 h at 4°C. The embryos were then washed three times in PBS for 10 min and incubated with the secondary antibody (chicken anti-mouse-alexa 488; 1:200; Invitrogen Molecular Probes, Eugene, OR, EUA), and goat anti-rabbit-alexa 555 (1:200; Invitrogen Molecular Probes, Eugene, OR, EUA) for 1 h. Nuclei were counterstained with 10 µL/mL Hoechst 33342 for 20 min. The embryos were washed three times for 10 min in PBS and examined under a fluorescence microscope. Reactions in which the primary antibody was omitted served as negative control. Images of each structure were captured with an AxioCam camera and stored using the AxioVision 4.7.1 software (Carl Zeiss, Jena, Germany).

Images were measured for fluorescence intensity on each blastomere (day 5 embryos) using Adobe Photoshop CS3 (Adobe Systems Inc., Beaverton, OR, USA). First, the three images from each embryo (HOECHST, Alexa 488 and Alexa 555) were placed together in a new file, in different layers. Nuclei were selected with the magic wand tool in HOECHST layer for each blastomere. Sections were measured using the histogram function through the red (H3k27me3) and green (H3k9ac) channels. Photoshop assigns intensity values between 0 and 255 to each pixel in the selected area and then averages these intensities, giving the mean intensity of the selected region. For each embryo, the mean intensity of blastomeres was normalized to the lowest level. After, levels were classified into 7 categories.

2.7 Statistical analysis

Mean frequency of each category of normalized blastomeres was analyzed by one-way ANOVA and means were compared by the Tukey test. Statistical analysis was performed using the SAS 9.1 software (SAS Institute Inc., Cary, NC, USA).

3. Results

We evaluated two replicates and 12 embryos during the transition from 8- to 16-cell stages, totaling 169 blastomeres. The pattern detected for each embryo can be seen in Figure 1. As we can observe, levels of H3k27me3 varied accordingly to levels of H3k9ac. In others words, blastomeres that presented higher H3k27me3 tended to present higher H3k9ac, which means that, for those embryos, global increases on repressive marks (H3k27me3) leads to increases in permissive marks (H3k9ac) as well.

Then we normalized the fluorescence level of each blastomere to the lowest level obtained, within each embryo. In this analysis, we observed that some embryos displayed a high individual variation between blastomeres, as demonstrated in Figure 2.

Therefore, we divided the embryos into two classes: A, for embryos that presented similar H3k9ac and H3k27me3 between blastomeres (8 embryos, 66%), and B, for embryos that exhibited variations between blastomeres (at least 2 blastomeres presenting 2fold increase in H3k9ac compared to the lowest blastomere) (4 embryos, 33%). Within each class, we classified the blastomeres accordingly to their intensity level: 1 to 1.5 (I), 1.5 to 2 (II), 2 to 2.5 (III), 2.5 to 3 (IV), 3 to 3.5 (V), 3.5 to 4 (VI), 4 to 4.5 (VII).

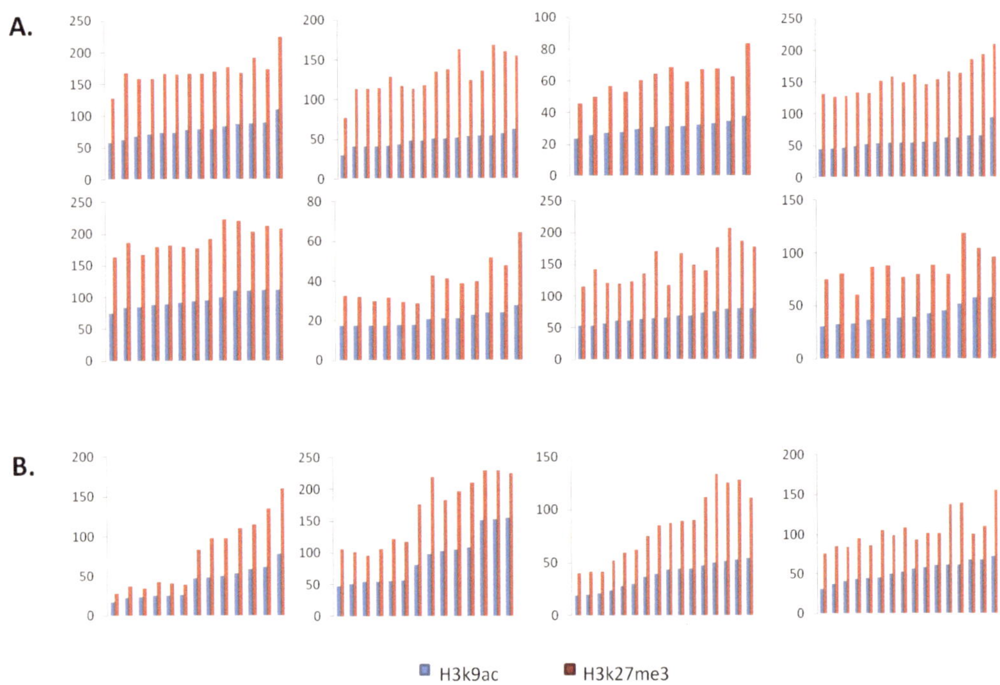

Fig. 1. Pattern of H3k9ac and H3k27me3 for 12 different embryos. Rows represent fluorescence levels of individual blastomeres. A) Embryos that presented similar levels of H3k9ac and H3k27me3 between blastomeres. B) Embryos that presented at least 2 blastomeres presenting 2-fold increases on H3k9ac levels, comparing to lowest level.

In class A embryos, we detected for H3k9ac a higher ($P < 0.05$) frequency of level I blastomeres, corresponding to 80%. The other blastomeres were classified in level II (18.3%) and III (1.6%). In this class of embryos, we did not detect any blastomeres in levels IV-VII, which means that most blastomeres presented similar lower levels of H3k9ac. The same pattern was observed in class I embryos for repressive mark H3k27me3. These results indicate that H3k9ac and H3k27me3 levels are constant between blastomeres in class I embryos, and their variation to the lowest blastomere level is only 2.5 fold maximum, in a small percentage of cells. Also, H3k9ac and H3k27me3 exhibited the same pattern of expression.

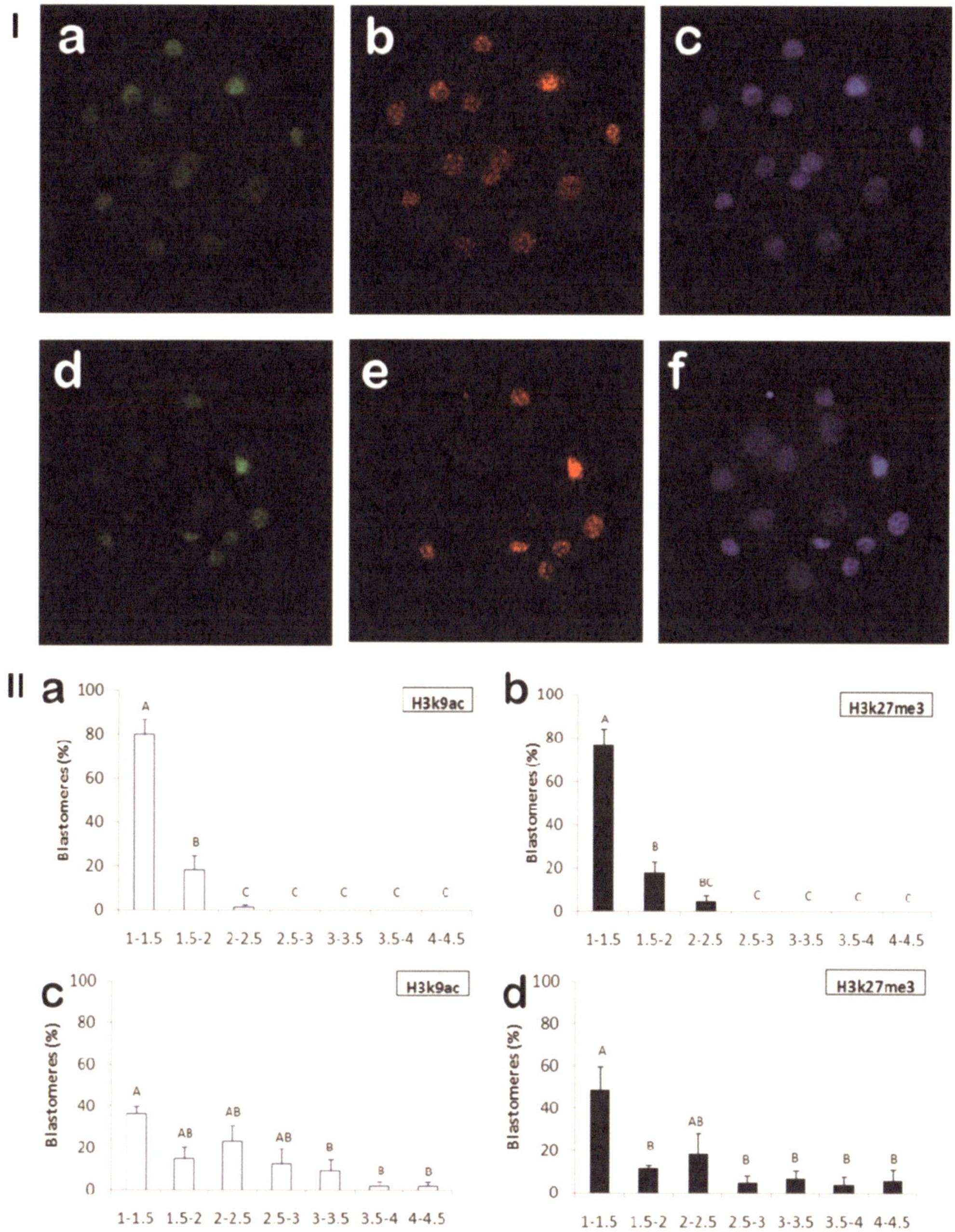

Fig. 2. Levels of H3k9ac and H3k27me3 in individual blastomeres from 12- to 16-cell embryos. I) Immunocitochemistry reaction for H3k9ac (Alexa 488, green) and H3k27me3 (Alexa 555, red) in class A (a,b) and class B (d,e) embryos. Nuclei were counterstained with HOECHST 33342 (c,f). II) Percentage (mean ± S.E.) of blastomeres from class A (a,b) and B (c,d) in H3k9ac and H3k27me3 level categories. In each embryo, blastomeres were normalized to the lowest H3k9ac level. [ABC]Means with different letters within the same group are not equal (ANOVA one way and Tukey post test, $P < 0.05$).

On the other hand, when we assessed class B embryos, we observed that only 36% blastomeres were classified as level I. This percentage was superior ($P < 0.05$) when compared to the percentage of embryos classified as levels V (9.2%), VI (1.9%) and VII (1.9%), but was similar to the frequency observed for levels II (14.8%), III (23.2%) and IV (12.4%). Thus, it can be suggested that a higher variation among H3k9ac levels is present in class B embryos. Additionally, for H3k27me3, the same pattern was observed, although level I frequency was higher (48.4%) and similar to level III (18.5%), and both levels I and III were superior ($P < 0.05$) to levels II (11.7%), IV (5.0%), V (6.6%), VI (3.8%) and VII (5.8%). Based on these results, it can be infered that, for class B embryos, levels of H3k9ac and H3k27me3 displayed a remarkable variation between blastomeres, up to 4.5 fold higher than the lowest blastomere level.

We also wanted, we wanted to confirm if the variations observed for H3k9ac and H3k27me3 were occuring in the same intense for both marks. Therefore, each blastomere level was tested for Person's correlation analysis. It was observed an extremely high correlation coeficient ($r = 0.913$) and a significant P value ($P < 0.0001$), confirming our hypothesis that H3k9ac and H3k27me3 are hightly correlated (Figure 3). In other words, we observed that in 12- to 16-cell embryos repressive and permissive marks vary in the same direction and intensity.

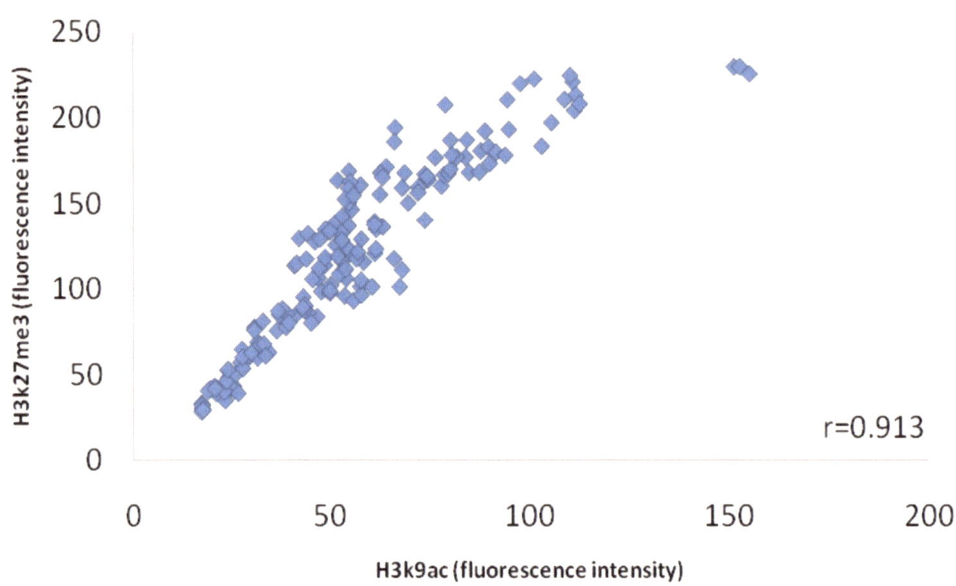

Fig. 3. Correlation between H3k9ac and H3k27me3 in individual blastomeres from 12- to 16-cell embryos.

4. Conclusions and future directions

Our results describe the presence of two distinguishable populations of bovine embryos during the 4th cell cycle, considering their epigenetic status. One population presented similar levels of repressive and permissive marks in all blastomeres, while the second one displayed a remarkable variation among their blastomeres.

Those changes were reported 2 cell cycles earlier than lineage specification in blastocysts. In mice, it has been demonstrated that differences in histone modifications between blastomeres as early as at the 4-cell stage reflect pluripotency, 2 cycles before trophectoderm differentiation (Torres-Padilla et al., 2007). Furthermore, only a specific population of embryos, based on their cleavage pattern, presented this difference in histone modification levels between blastomeres. Therefore, it is possible that the same phenomena happens in bovine embryos, and that might explain our findings.

In other words, those variable histone modification levels within class B embryos might show differences in pluripotent competence between blastomeres in the same embryo. In this case, cellular differentiation, which can be clearly seen after blastocyst formation, might have already been initiated in the 16-cell bovine embryo. However, this preliminary data should be further investigated. Time lapse studies, following the cell fate decisions of those blastomeres and better characterization of how they were derived are needed to elucidate this question.

In addition, here we demonstrated that global levels of permissive and repressive marks are correlated at this time point. These results suggest that, in 4th cell cycle embryos, no global switch between repressive and permissive marks is detected; and that level of those marks still goes along together.

In conclusion, embryonic genome activation is a crucial step across early embryo development, and it is accompanied by a dramatic change in epigenetic profile of blastomeres. Monitoring of histone modifications related to euchromatin and heterochromatin is an important tool to assess developmental competence in a sense that those marks are altered when manipulation and environmental stress conditions are applied. In this chapter, we described the pattern of IVC embryos in the cycle after embryonic genome activation, considering a repressive (H3k27me3) and a permissive (H3k9ac) histone modification mark. Those experiments would also be useful in order to compare culture conditions of IVF embryos, and how they would respond after environmental challenges. Interestingly, we found two distinguishable populations of embryos, one presenting similar profiles between blastomeres and other presenting remarkable changes between blastomeres. This observation should be further studied, as it might be reflecting distinct cleavage pattern embryos and pluripotency competence.

5. Acknowledgment

The authors are grateful to FAPESP for the financial support provided.

6. References

Adenot, P.G.; Mercier, Y.; Renard, J.P. & Thompson, E.M. (1997). Differential h4 acetylation of paternal and maternal chromatin precedes DNA replication and differential transcriptional activity in pronuclei of 1-cell mouse embryos. *Development,* Vol.124, No.22, (November 1997), pp. 4615-4625, ISSN 0950-1991

Aoki, F.; Worrad, D.M. & Schultz, R.M. (1997). Regulation of transcriptional activity during the first and second cell cycles in the preimplantation mouse embryo. *Developmental Biology,* Vol.181, No.2, (January 1997), pp. 296-307, ISSN 0012-1606

Artley, J.K.; Braude, P.R. & Johnson, M.H. (1992). Gene activity and cleavage arrest in human pre-embryos. *Human Reproduction,* Vol.7, No.7, (August 1992), pp. 1014-1021, ISSN 0268-1161

Badr, H.; Bongioni, G.; Abdoon, A.S.; Kandil, O. & Puglisi, R. (2007). Gene expression in the in vitro-produced preimplantation bovine embryos. *Zygote,* Vol.15, No.4, (November 2007), pp. 355-367, ISSN 0967-1994

Bannister, A.J. & Kouzarides, T. (2011). Regulation of chromatin by histone modifications. *Cell Research,* Vol.21, No.3, (March 2011), pp. 381-395, ISSN 1748-7838

Bensaude, O.; Babinet, C.; Morange, M. & Jacob, F. (1983). Heat shock proteins, first major products of zygotic gene activity in mouse embryo. *Nature,* Vol.305, No.5932, (September 1983), pp. 331-333, ISSN 0028-0836

Bertolini, M.; Mason, J.B.; Beam, S.W.; Carneiro, G.F.; Sween, M.L.; Kominek, D.J.; Moyer, A.L.; Famula, T.R.; Sainz, R.D. & Anderson, G.B. (2002). Morphology and morphometry of in vivo- and in vitro-produced bovine concepti from early pregnancy to term and association with high birth weights. *Theriogenology,* Vol.58, No.5, (September 2002), pp. 973-994, ISSN 0093-691X

Bolton, V.; Wren, M. & Parsons, J. (1991). Pregnancies after invitro fertilization and transfer of human blastocysts. *Fertility and Sterility,* Vol.55, No.4, (April 1991), pp. 830-832, ISSN 0015-0282

Braude, P.; Bolton, V. & Moore, S. (1988). Human gene expression first occurs between the four- and eight-cell stages of preimplantation development. *Nature,* Vol.332, No.6163, (March 1988), pp. 459-461, ISSN 0028-0836

Brinsko, S.P.; Ball, B.A.; Ignotz, G.G.; Thomas, P.G.; Currie, W.B. & Ellington, J.E. (1995). Initiation of transcription and nucleologenesis in equine embryos. *Molecular Reproduction and Development,* Vol.42, No.3, (November 1995), pp. 298-302, ISSN 1040-452X

Brunet-Simon, A.; Henrion, G.; Renard, J.P. & Duranthon, V. (2001). Onset of zygotic transcription and maternal transcript legacy in the rabbit embryo. *Molecular Reproduction and Development,* Vol.58, No.2, (February 2001), pp. 127-136, ISSN 1040-452X

Crosby, I.M.; Gandolfi, F. & Moor, R.M. (1988). Control of protein synthesis during early cleavage of sheep embryos. *Journal of Reproduction and Fertility,* Vol.82, No.2, (March 1988), pp. 769-775, ISSN 0022-4251

Davis, W. & Schultz, R.M. (1997). Role of the first round of DNA replication in reprogramming gene expression in the preimplantation mouse embryo. *Molecular Reproduction and Development,* Vol.47, No.4, (August 1997), pp. 430-434, ISSN 1040-452X

De Sousa, P.A.; Watson, A.J. & Schultz, R.M. (1998). Transient expression of a translation initiation factor is conservatively associated with embryonic gene activation in murine and bovine embryos. *Biology of Reproduction,* Vol.59, No.4, (October 1998), pp. 969-977, ISSN 0006-3363

Dean, W.; Santos, F. & Reik, W. (2003). Epigenetic reprogramming in early mammalian development and following somatic nuclear transfer. *Seminars in Cell and Developmental Biology,* Vol.14, No.1, (February 2003), pp. 93-100, ISSN 1084-9521

Dobson, A.T.; Raja, R.; Abeyta, M.J.; Taylor, T.; Shen, S.; Haqq, C. & Pera, R.A. (2004). The unique transcriptome through day 3 of human preimplantation development. *Human Molecular Genetics,* Vol.13, No.14, (July 2004), pp. 1461-1470, ISSN 0964-6906

Enright, B.P.; Jeong, B.S.; Yang, X. & Tian, X.C. (2003). Epigenetic characteristics of bovine donor cells for nuclear transfer: Levels of histone acetylation. *Biology of Reproduction,* Vol.69, No.5, (November 2003), pp. 1525-1530, ISSN 0006-3363

Hamatani, T.; Carter, M.G.; Sharov, A.A. & Ko, M.S. (2004). Dynamics of global gene expression changes during mouse preimplantation development. *Developmental Cell,* Vol.6, No.1, (January 2004), pp. 117-131, ISSN 1534-5807

Hamatani, T.; Ko, M.S.H.; Yamada, M.; Kuji, N.; Mizusawa, Y.; Shoji, M.; Hada, T.; Asada, H.; Maruyama, T. & Yoshimura, Y. (2006). Global gene expression profiling of preimplantation embryos. *Human Cell,* Vol.19, No.3, (August 2006), pp. 98-117, ISSN 0914-7470

Hardy, K.; Handyside, A. & Winston, R. (1989). The human blastocyst: cell number, death and allocation during late preimplantation development in vitro. *Development,* Vol.107, No.3, (November 1989), pp. (597-604), ISSN 0950-1991

Kang, Y.K.; Park, J.S.; Koo, D.B.; Choi, Y.H.; Kim, S.U.; Lee, K.K. & Han, Y.M. (2002). Limited demethylation leaves mosaic-type methylation states in cloned bovine pre-implantation embryos. *The EMBO Journal,* Vol.21, No.5, (March 2002), pp. 1092-1000, ISSN 0261-4189

Kim, J.M.; Liu, H.; Tazaki, M.; Nagata, M. & Aoki, F. (2003). Changes in histone acetylation during mouse oocyte meiosis. *Journal of Cell Biolology,* Vol.162, No.1, (July 2003), pp. 37-46, ISSN 0021-9525

Kouzarides, T. (2007). Chromatin modifications and their function. *The Cell,* Vol.128, No.4, (February 2007), pp. 693-705, ISSN 0092-8674

Li, E. (2002). Chromatin modification and epigenetic reprogramming in mammalian development. *Nature Reviews Genetics,* Vol.3, No.9, (September 2002), pp. 662-673, ISSN 1471-0056

Lonergan, P.; Rizos, D.; Gutierrez-Adan, A.; Fair, T. & Boland, M.P. (2003). Oocyte and embryo quality: Effect of origin, culture conditions and gene expression patterns. *Reproduction in Domestic Animals,* Vol.38, No.4, (August 2003), pp. 259-267, ISSN 0936-6768

Maalouf, W.E.; Alberio, R. & Campbell, K.H. (2008). Differential acetylation of histone h4 lysine during development of in vitro fertilized, cloned and parthenogenetically activated bovine embryos. *Epigenetics,* Vol.3, No.4, (July - August 2008), pp. 199-209, ISSN 1559-2308

Martin, C. & Zhang, Y. (2005). The diverse functions of histone lysine methylation. *Nature Reviews Molecular Cell Biology,* Vol.6, No.11, (November 2005), pp. 838-849, ISSN 1471-0072

Mcgraw, S.; Robert, C.; Massicotte, L. & Sirard, M.A. (2003). Quantification of histone acetyltransferase and histone deacetylase transcripts during early bovine embryo development. *Biology of Reproduction,* Vol.68, No.2, (February 2003), pp. (383-389), ISSN 0006-3363

Meirelles, F.V.; Caetano, A.R.; Watanabe, Y.F.; Ripamonte, P.; Carambula, S.F.; Merighe, G.K. & Garcia, S.M. (2004). Genome activation and developmental block in bovine embryos. *Animal Reproduction Science,* Vol.82-83, (July 2004), pp. 13-20, ISSN 0378-4320

Moore, G.P. (1975). The rna polymerase activity of the preimplantation mouse embryo. *Journal of Embryology & Experimental Morphology,* Vol.34, No.2, (October 1975), pp. 291-298, ISSN 0022-0752

Nothias, J.Y.; Miranda, M. & Depamphilis, M.L. (1996). Uncoupling of transcription and translation during zygotic gene activation in the mouse. *The EMBO Journal,* Vol.15, No.20, (October 1996), pp. 5715-5725, ISSN 0261-4189

Oliveira, C.S.; Saraiva, N.Z.; De Souza, M.M.; Tetzner TAD; De Lima, M.R. & Garcia, J.M. (2010). Effects of histone hyperacetylation on the preimplantation development of male and female bovine embryos. *Reproduction, Fertility and Development,* Vol.22, No.6 (2010), pp. (1041-1048), ISSN 1031-3613

Oliveira, C.S.; Saraiva, N.Z.; De Souza, M.M.; De Almeida Drummond Tetzner TAD; De Lima, M.R. & Garcia, J.M. (2011). Supplementation with the histone deacetylase inhibitor trichostatin a during in vitro culture of bovine embryos. *Zygote,* Vol.26 (August 2011), pp. 1-5, ISSN 1469-8730

Rambhatla, L. & Latham, K.E. (1995). Strain-specific progression of alpha-amanitin-treated mouse embryos beyond the two-cell stage. *Molecular Reproduction and Development,* Vol.41, No.1, (May 1995), pp. 16-19, ISSN 1040-452X

Reik, W.; Santos, F. & Dean, W. (2003). Mammalian epigenomics: Reprogramming the genome for development and therapy. *Theriogenology,* Vol.59, No.1, (January 2003), pp. 21-32, ISSN 0093-691X

Rizos, D.; Lonergan, P.; Boland, M.P.; Arroyo-García, R.; Pintado, B.; De La Fuente, J. & Gutiérrez-Adán, A. (2002). Analysis of differential messenger rna expression between bovine blastocysts produced in different culture systems: Implications for blastocyst quality. *Biology of Reproduction,* Vol.66, No.3, (March 2002), pp. 589-595, ISSN 0006-3363

Santos, F.; Zakhartchenko, V.; Stojkovic, M.; Peters, A.; Jenuwein, T.; Wolf, E.; Reik, W. & Dean, W. (2003). Epigenetic marking correlates with developmental potential in cloned bovine preimplantation embryos. *Current Biology,* Vol.13, No.13, (July 2003), pp. 1116-1121, ISSN 0960-9822

Sanz, L.A.; Kota, S.K. & Feil, R. (2010). Genome-wide DNA demethylation in mammals. *Genome Biology,* Vol.11, No.3, (2010), pp. 110, ISSN 1465-6914

Sarmento, O.F.; Digilio, L.C.; Wang, Y.; Perlin, J.; Herr, J.C.; Allis, C.D. & Coonrod, S.A. (2004). Dynamic alterations of specific histone modifications during early murine development. *Journal of Cell Science,* Vol.117, No.19, (September 2004), pp. 4449-4459, ISSN 0021-9533

Schramm, R.D. & Bavister, B.D. (1999). Onset of nucleolar and extranucleolar transcription and expression of fibrillarin in macaque embryos developing in vitro. *Biology of Reproduction,* Vol.60, No.3, (March 1999), pp. (721-728), ISSN 0006-3363

Schultz, R.M. (2002). The molecular foundations of the maternal to zygotic transition in the preimplantation embryo. *Human Reproduction Update,* Vol.8, No.4, (July - August, 2002), pp. 323-331, ISSN 1355-4786

Sepulveda, S.; Portella, J.; Noriega, L.; Escudero, E. & Noriega, L. (2011). Extended culture up to the blastocyst stage: A strategy to avoid multiple pregnancies in assisted reproductive technologies. *Biological Research,* Vol.44, No.2, (2011,2011), pp. 195-199, ISSN 0716-9760

Shire, J.G. & Whitten, W.K. (1980). Genetic variation in the timing of first cleavage in mice: Effect of maternal genotype. *Biology of Reproduction,* Vol.23, No.2, (September 1980), pp. 369-376, ISSN 0006-3363

Spinaci, M., Seren, E. & Mattioli, M. (2004). Maternal chromatin remodeling during maturation and after fertilization in mouse oocytes. *Molecular Reproduction and Development,* Vol.69, No.2, (October 2004), pp. 215-221, ISSN 1040-452X

Tesarík, J.; Kopecný, V.; Plachot, M. & Mandelbaum, J. (1988). Early morphological signs of embryonic genome expression in human preimplantation development as revealed by quantitative electron microscopy. *Developmental Biology,* Vol.128, No.1, (July 1988), pp. 15-20, ISSN 0012-1606

Torres-Padilla, M.E.; Parfitt, D.E.; Kouzarides, T. & Zernicka-Goetz, M. (2007). Histone arginine methylation regulates pluripotency in the early mouse embryo. *Nature,* Vol.445, No.7124, (January 2007), pp. 214-218, ISSN 1476-4687

Vassena, R.; Boué, S.; González-Roca, E.; Aran, B.; Auer, H.; Veiga, A. & Belmonte, J.C. (2011). Waves of early transcriptional activation and pluripotency program initiation during human preimplantation development. *Development,* Vol.138, No.17, (September 2011), pp. 3699-3709, ISSN 1477-9129

Wolffe, A.P. & Guschin, D. (2000). Review: Chromatin structural features and targets that regulate transcription. *Journal of Structural Biology,* Vol.129, No.2-3, (April 2000), pp. 102-122, ISSN 1047-8477

Wrenzycki, C.; Herrmann, D.; Carnwath, J.W. & Niemann, H. (1996). Expression of the gap junction gene connexin43 (cx43) in preimplantation bovine embryos derived in vitro or in vivo. *Journal of Reproduction and Fertility,* Vol.108, No.1, (September 1996), pp. 17-24, ISSN 0022-4251

Wrenzycki, C.; Lucas-Hahn, A.; Herrmann, D.; Lemme, E.; Korsawe, K. & Niemann, H. Compensation of the x-linked gene transcripts g6pd, pgk, and xist in preimplantation bovine embryos. *Biology of Reproduction,* Vol.66, No.1, (January 2002), pp. 127-134), ISSN 0006-3363

Wrenzycki, C.; Herrmann, D.; Lucas-Hahn, A.; Lemme, E.; Korsawe, K. & Niemann, H. (2004). Gene expression patterns in in vitro-produced and somatic nuclear transfer-derived preimplantation bovine embryos: Relationship to the large offspring syndrome? *Animal Reproduction Science,* Vol.82-83, (July 2004), pp. 593-603, ISSN 0378-4320

Zhang, J.; Li, X.; Peng, Y.; Guo, X.; Heng, B. & Tong, G. (2010). Reduction in exposure of human embryos outside the incubator enhances embryo quality and blastulation rate. *Reproductive Biomedicine Online,* Vol.20, No.4, (April 2010), pp. 510-515, ISSN 1472-6483

6

Safety in Assisted Reproductive Technologies: Insights from Gene Expression Studies During Preimplantation Development

Daniela Bebbere, Luisa Bogliolo,
Federica Ariu, Irma Rosati and Sergio Ledda
*Department of Veterinary Clinics and Pathology,
University of Sassari,
Italy*

1. Introduction

The mammalian oocyte and embryo display considerable plasticity. Even in sub-optimal conditions, as in vitro environment may be certainly considered, the oocyte is able to mature, face fertilization and develop first into an embryo and finally to a live offspring. Such ability has encouraged, over the decades, the development of numerous in vitro assisted reproductive technologies (ART) in several species, included human. Nowadays, more than 30 years after its inception, human ART are routinely and successfully applied to solve fertility problems, which affect ~ 15% of reproductive age couples and have significant medical, social and financial implications.

The use of ART has increased steadily over the last years also because of its perceived safety. Worldwide, it is now estimated that more than 3 million babies have been born as a consequence of the application of ART (Grace & Sinclair, 2009). Although the majority of children born after ART are healthy, safety is still a cornerstone for reproductive technologies.

A number of studies have hypothesized that manipulation of conception may negatively affect embryonic and fetal development and possibly have lifelong consequences on the offspring (DeRyche et al., 2002; Thompson et al., 2002). Moreover, abundant evidence from animal species showed that in vitro manipulation during ART influences the genetics and physiologic development of the embryos.

These data support the idea that the earliest stages of life set the basis for the future health of the offspring (Barker, 1997) and highlight an inadequate understanding of the cellular and molecular basis of reproduction. A deeper knowledge about preimplantation development is a fundamental prerequisite for a safer application of reproductive in vitro technologies.

Because of the peculiar characteristics of the mammalian oocyte and pre-implantation embryo, the analysis of gene expression status during the very first phases of life is essential for the evaluation of ART safety. As a matter of fact, disruption in the regulation of gene expression has been often observed as a consequence of in vitro manipulation (Humpherys et al., 2001; Yang et al., 2005; Young et al., 2001).

Importantly, in several species ART has been associated with imprinting disruption. In vitro culture was seen to cause abnormal epigenetic modifications and subsequent deregulation of imprinted genes, in association with early embryonic losses and a variety of abnormal phenotypes (de Sousa et al., 2001; Wrenzycki & Niemann, 2003; Yang et al., 2005; Young et al., 2001). Faulty nuclear reprogramming is considered the primary cause of the reported defects.

Epidemiologic studies have revealed that the use of some reproductive technologies is associated with an increased frequency of imprinting defects in humans as well (De Rycke et al., 2002; Powell, 2003; Stromberg et al., 2002; Thompson et al., 2002). Disruption of imprinting has raised particular concern since it is involved in the etiology of severe developmental disorders in humans (Arnaud & Feil, 2005; Scarano et al., 2005), such as Beckwith-Wiedemann and Angelman syndromes.

Studies on preimplantation embryo development are crucial to gain insight into the molecular mechanisms correlated with an undisturbed embryonic and fetal development and to improve efficiency and safety of assisted reproductive biotechnologies.

Due to the obvious scarcity of human oocytes and embryos for research, the use of appropriate animals models (reliable, cost-effective and featuring the characteristics of human fertilization) is of irreplaceable support.

In this chapter, we will discuss the effect of ART on early embryonic development, focusing on gene expression. The characteristics of the transcriptome of mammalian oocytes and pre-implantation embryos will be described, as well as the reprogramming events that take place during oocyte-to-embryo transition. The effects of ART on regulation of gene expression and on imprinting will be examined, together with short- and long-term consequences for the embryo/fetus/offspring. The benefits of using animal models will be addressed, highlighting the peculiarities and advantages of different mammalian species.

2. Controversy on safety in assisted reproduction

Since the birth of the first baby conceived by in vitro fertilization, in 1978 (Steptoe & Edwards, 1978), more than 3 million babies have been born as a consequence of ART application (Grace & Sinclair, 2009). The original IVF technique, which involved mixing oocytes and sperm in vitro and then transferring the embryo into the womb, was evaluated as "safe" in follow-up studies of IVF children (Friedler et al., 1992; Saunders & Lancaster, 1989). Progressively more interventionist and daring techniques have been set up to treat infertility. Women were hormonally treated to stimulate ovulation, oocytes and sperm have been manipulated in various way to achieve fertilization, microassisted techniques, such as Intracytoplasmic Sperm Injection (ICSI) and pre-implantation genetic diagnosis (PGD), were developed. However, unlike most therapeutic procedures used in medicine, assisted reproductive technologies never underwent rigorous safety testing before clinical use. Consequently, safety concerns arise for at least two major reasons:

i. treatments for infertility overcome natural barriers that prevent fertilization. (i.e. as these technologies are used to overcome infertility phenotypes that may have a genetic basis, unwanted genetic traits may be possibly transmitted to offspring)
ii. the reproductive technology itself may exert adverse consequences on the health of the offspring.

The application of IVF/ICSI to treat infertility is a clear example of this phenomenon. ICSI is an in vitro fertilization procedure in which a single sperm is injected directly into an oocyte. It was developed in 1992 (Palermo et al., 1992) and was quickly undertaken as allows men not producing healthy mobile sperm to become fathers. Nowadays, ICSI is often the method of choice for ART, and accounts for more than half of all assisted reproductive treatment in the western countries (USA 57.5%, Australia/New Zealand 58.6%, Europe 59.3%; Andersen et al., 2008). The use of such an aggressive technique has raised heavy concerns. The injection of the sperm directly inside the oocyte bypasses natural selection mechanisms, possibly passing infertility problems to the next generation or, even worse, overcoming natural barriers that are meant to stop genetic abnormalities carried out by faulty sperms. Moreover, ICSI may physically impair molecular mechanisms needed for proper fertilization and further development.

The concern about ART safety is supported by several studies that assessed the risk of birth defects in children conceived by ART compared to naturally conceived infants.

Higher risk of birth defects was reported in children conceived by IVF or ICSI compared to controls (Allen et al., 2006; Hansen et al., 2002; Kurinczuk & Bower, 1997), while singletons conceived after assisted fertilization consistently showed higher risk of low birthweight, preterm delivery and perinatal death than spontaneously conceived singletons (Allen et al., 2006; Bergh et al., 1999; Jackson et al., 2004; McDonald et al., 2005, 2009; McGovern et al., 2004; Schieve et al., 2002; Sutcliff & Ludwig, 2007;). Noticeably, even after adjusting for factors such as multiple birth, mother's age and preterm deliveries, the risks of birth defects highlighted in these studies remain higher for assisted reproduction-groups.

Over the years, this scientific evidence on ART safety has attracted considerable attention and has been highly criticized, especially by practitioners of assisted reproduction. The studies were accused of design flows, including the retrospective nature of most of them. In addition, the debate was enlivened by several studies clashing with the evidence of safety risks associated with ART procedures: no evidence for worries in IVF/ICSI babies was in fact repeatedly reported (Bonduelle et al., 1996; Romundstad et al., 2008).

It has been argued that some of the morbidity associated with ART does not result from the techniques, but from the underlying health risks of being subfertile. A large population-based cohort study was carried out using sibling-relationship comparisons (women conceiving at least one child spontaneously and one after ART; Romundstad et al., 2008). Results suggested that the adverse outcomes of assisted fertilisation compared with those in the general population could be due to factors leading to infertility, rather than factors related to the reproductive technology. Accordingly, studies of couples with reduced fertility, who eventually conceived spontaneously, showed higher risk of adverse perinatal outcomes than those without fertility problems (Basso & Baird, 2003; Draper et al., 1999; Ghazi et al., 1991; Henriksen et al., 1997; Williams et al., 1991).

In the bargain, the disagreement among studies is often due to different definition of "birth defects", leading to an inconsistent classification of congenital abnormalities and other adverse outcomes.

In summary, despite the large effort to study the effects of reproductive technologies, there is still only an incomplete picture of the risks associated with the use of ART. The existing worries on potential unpleasant outcomes on a short- and long-term call for increased studies on the basic biology of fertilization and pre-implantation development, and on the effect of in vitro manipulation of oocytes and embryos.

Research in animal models, which is by its nature free of the biases that make the studies in human defective, should be broadened to identify the potential risks of ART application on short and long-term.

3. Focus on preimplantation embryo development

It is nowadays accepted that the earliest stages of life set the basis for the future health of the offspring (Barker, 1997). From this perspective, it is foreseeable that any disturbance during the very early development, as well as sub-optimal conditions (i.e. in vitro environment), may adversely affect the future offspring. Accordingly, abundant evidence in several species assessed that manipulation of gametes and embryo through ART may exert undesirable consequences on the offspring on a short- and long-term (DeRyche et al., 2002; Thompson et al., 2002).

Although the use of fertility treatment is increasing all over the world and in vitro reproductive technologies are routinely applied in several species for both research and commercial purposes, the technologies are still far from being perfect. Even in the best cases, in vitro embryo production achieves success rates hardly comparable to the in vivo ones, indicating that current in vitro procedures do not sufficiently resemble the reproductive physiology. At the same time, ART conceived offspring was seen to be different from naturally conceived individuals. Further research on gametes and preimplantation embryos is therefore fundamental to ameliorate the technologies and to evaluate the effect on the offspring.

As transcription is the first biologic/adaptive response to a perturbation or to an external stimulus, an adequate understanding of the gene expression status and regulation during the very first phases of development is an essential approach for the evaluation of ART safety. For this reason, in recent years gene expression studies have been increasing and integrated the numerous experimental approaches used in the past. Although the birth of a live and healthy offspring is considered the best parameter to evaluate the fitness of an embryo, gene expression studies during pre-implantation development have the advantage of being cost- and time-effective and, most importantly, they highlight differences at the molecular level that may be undetectable at birth, but affect the health of the adult.

3.1 Transcriptome of mammalian oocytes and pre-implantation embryos

In mammals, oogenesis is characterized by alternating active meiotic progression to long times of meiotic arrest. Resumption of meiosis occurs in fully grown oocytes (FGO) that complete first meiosis and then mature to metaphase II (MII). Completion of meiosis is dependent on fertilization, that leads to anaphase II and the formation of the first mitotic interphase. The time from fertilization to implantation of the embryo in the uterus is called pre-implantation embryonic development (PED).

The regulation of gene expression in oocytes and pre-implantation embryos shows peculiar characteristics. Oocyte maturation and early pre-implantation development are essentially under "maternal command" from factors deposited in the cytoplasm during oocyte growth, independent of de novo transcription from the mature oocyte and the nascent embryo. The FGO contains all the maternal RNAs and proteins necessary to activate the molecular pathways required for fertilization and early embryogenesis (Cui and Kim, 2007; Pennetier et al., 2004). As a consequence, just after fertilization, the transcriptome of the embryo consists only in the maternally deposited transcripts. After several cell divisions, these maternal transcripts are specifically degraded and are replaced by embryonic transcripts produced by the new diploid cells, containing both maternal and paternal genes. This transition is termed embryo genome activation (EGA). The timing of EGA varies among species: in humans and bovines it occurs between the four- and eight- cell stages (Telford et al., 1990), in ovine between the eight-and the sixteen-cell stage (Kopecny, 1989), while in mouse between the one- and two-cell stage of development (Schultz, 1993).

Precise control of the dynamic changes that occur in the ooplasm during the phases of oocyte-to-embryo transition (OET), until EGA, is crucial for a proper development of the nascent embryo. The transcriptional quiescence requires extensive post-transcriptional and post-translational activities (Seydoux, 1996; Solter et al., 2002). Three major mechanisms take place, commencing at oocyte maturation and during the subsequent transcriptionally silent stages of development: (i) timely translation of stored maternal transcripts (ii) post-translational modification of existing and/or newly synthesized proteins (iii) degradation of no longer needed proteins and mRNAs.

These mechanisms exploit the differential stability of the maternal mRNAs stored in the ooplasm (Oh et al., 2000). During oocyte growth, many transcribed mRNAs are de-adenylated and stored in the ooplasm in a stable dormant form for subsequent translation. During translational activation, their limited 3' poly(A) tails lengthen (Bachvarova, 1992), a sign that active translation is occurring (Richter, 1999). Half of the poly(A) mRNAs found in the fully-grown oocyte is de-adenylated during maturation, and by the 2-cell stage, the embryo contains less than 30% original amount of adenylated mRNAs found in the egg (Piko & Clegg, 1982).

4. Animal models: Peculiarities and advantages of different mammalian species

Due to the obvious scarcity of human oocytes and embryos for research, the use of appropriate animals models is of irreplaceable support for studying the basic biology of fertilization and pre-implantation development and for ART optimization. This is possible because the molecular mechanisms contributing to oogenesis and to PED progression are highly conserved among mammals (Gilbert, 2000). Although EGA occurs at different stages of development in different mammalian species (Kopecny, 1989; Schultz, 1993; Telford et al., 1990), the mechanisms of activation of the embryonic genome are in fact similar. All mammalian species progress through the same morphologic stages; perhaps, the most marked difference is the amount of time spent at each step, while the other notable interspecies differences appear after the blastocyst stage.

The comparison between maternally-deposited and EGA-activated transcripts in humans, cattle and mice indicates that maternal transcripts are generally more conserved than transcripts newly synthesized by the embryo (Xie et al., 2010). The conservation of the first phases of PED among mammals has encouraged the use of animal models for studying meiotic progression and early pre-implantation development. Indeed, most knowledge about maternal translation and embryonic transcription reprogramming is based on mouse (Hamatani et al., 2004; Pangas et al., 2006; Xie et al., 2010) or ruminant models (Misirlioglu et al., 2006; Vigneault et al., 2009a, 2009b; Xie et al., 2010), while limited data are available from primates and humans (Nyholt de Prada et al., 2010; Xie et al., 2010; Zhang et al., 2009a, 2009b).

The main features sought in animal models are reliability, cost-effectiveness and biologic similarity to human fertilization. Each mammalian species exhibits specific characteristics and advantages for reproductive studies. Combining information related to a specific reproductive issue in different animal models has proved to be a useful approach to identify conserved mechanisms (Xie et al., 2010). Moreover, unveiling the basis of species-specific responses to certain technologies contributes to identifying the molecular or cellular mechanisms solicited by the manipulation.

Rodents, such as rats and mice, have been widely used and have yielded fundamental contributions to biomedical research. Over the past century, the mouse has developed into the premier mammalian model system for genetic research. Genetic and physiological similarities to humans allowed the generation of disease and treatment models and the creation of specific mutant lineages. The advantages of mouse as a model for human medicine include the genetic and physiological similarities to humans, the relatively low cost of maintenance, its ability to quickly multiply, as well as the ease with which its genome can be manipulated and analyzed.

The contributions of mouse model to understanding reproductive processes are numerous. Functional studies in mouse paved the way to the discovery of maternal effect genes (MEG) in mammals (Dade et al., 2004; Dean, 2002; Rajkovic & Matzuk, 2002). These oocyte specific genes, stored in the growing oocyte, are involved in the regulation of early cleavage, and their knockout often results in the inability of the embryo to develop beyond the first cleavage. *Zar1, MATER, NPM2,* are among the MEG that were later seen to be conserved in all the studied mammalian species, as bovine (Pennetier et al., 2004; Thelie et al., 2007; Uzbekova et al., 2006), human (Tong et al., 2002; Uzbekova et al., 2006; Wu et al., 2003b), swine (Uzbekova et al., 2006) and sheep (Bebbere et al., 2008).

While the mouse is an ideal model to study knockout effects and to create specific mutant lineages, large domestic animals are more suitable to study different aspects of reproduction. Sheep and cattle are mono-ovular and have similar reproductive endocrinology and ovarian biology (Gosden et al., 1994). They display biparentally contributed assembly of the zygotic centrosome during fertilization, like humans, while rodents show maternal inheritance. In ruminants, EGA occurs during the period from 4- to -16 cell stage (Camous, 1986; Kopecny, 1989), encompassing the period when it occurs in humans (Telford et al., 1990). Conversely, in mice EGA occurs very early and abruptly at the 2-cell stage, thus narrowing the window of opportunity for analysis of the reprogramming events during this delicate phase. The spreading of EGA over 3 to 4 cell cycles in large domestic animals allows a better analysis of the progressive phases leading to the major wave of transcriptional activation (Bensaude & Morange, 1983). This feature allowed the identification of functions specific to different points of PED, and was exploited in the analysis of MEG expression in sheep (Bebbere et al., 2008) and cattle (Bettegowda et al., 2007; Pennetier et al., 2004, 2006).

Research on ruminants is favored by the large numbers of gametes that can be easily obtained from farms and slaughterhouses. Moreover, the detailed information on ruminant fertilization is strengthened by years of research and well-defined reproductive technology aimed at increasing the productivity of farm animals. Several reproductive technologies have been developed in farm species, but have then contributed to human reproductive medicine and to understanding reproductive processes. Artificial insemination (Herman, 1981), semen cryopreservation (Foote, 1982; Polge, 1949), superovulation, in vitro fertilization and embryo transfer are among the many techniques that were mainly developed in farm animals (Roberts, 2001).

5. The effects of ART on regulation of gene expression: Pros or cons?

Embryonic development in vitro may be compromised by inappropriate in vitro culture systems designed to induce oocyte maturation or to sustain fertilization and further development. Media used for in vitro oocyte and embryo culture, being so far based more on empiricism than on precise knowledge of embryo needs, inevitably provide a variety of discordant biochemical signals that confound the reprogramming of at least some embryos. The sub-acute nature of some alterations induced by in vitro embryo production may remain undetected in the short term. Embryos are often capable to reach the blastocyst stage, a frequently used hallmark for the efficiency of in vitro embryo culture systems, in spite of a sub-optimal culture environment. Such ability, however, may be inconvenient for their postnatal health. Studies in several mammalian species have indeed shown that in vitro conditions during PED do affect the quality of the embryo, albeit being compatible with full-term development.

Abundant evidence based on different systems to evaluate embryo quality showed that in vitro-produced embryos are not necessarily similar to naturally conceived ones and it is now widely accepted that embryos derived from in vitro culture are of inferior quality to those derived in vivo. Compared to their in vivo counterparts, IVP embryos display a number of marked differences, e.g., gross morphology (color, density, cell number and size), timing of development (Greve et al., 1995), zona pellucida stability and resistance to criopreservation (Leibo & Loskutoff, 1993; Niemann et al., 1995).

The proliferation of molecular technologies has given a boost to experimentation and confirmed that in vitro environment does alter the oocyte and early embryo molecular structure (Ecker et al., 2004; Gutiérrez-Adán et al., 2004; Lonergan et al., 2003a, 2003b; McEvoy et al., 2001; Niemann et al., 2000; Summers & Biggers, 2003). In particular, the analysis of gene expression evidenced that the differences in phenotype correspond to altered transcriptomes in the developing embryos, and gave for the first time the opportunity to identify the single molecules solicited by in vitro environment.

Many studies examined the differences in the expression of specific genes, selected on a functional basis, between in vitro- and in vivo produced embryos of several species (Corcoran et al., 2007; Knijn et al., 2005; Rizos et al., 2002a). The expression of laminin chain-specific genes (Shim et al., 1996) and of gap junction gene Cx43 (Wrenzycki et al., 1996) was seen to decrease in in vitro produced blastocysts, while expression of stress-related genes, such as Heat Shock Protein 70.1, was seen to increase in pre-implantation embryos due to in vitro exposure (Christians et al., 1995). Genes related to glucose metabolism were seen to be down-regulated in IVP embryos (Knijn et al., 2005; Uechi et al., 1997; Wrenzycki et al., 1998a). A temporal variation in several transcript abundance was observed in embryos at different stages of PED cultured in vitro or in vivo (Corcoran et al., 2007; Tesfaye et al., 2004).

The advent of microarray technologies offered the opportunity to gain an insight into the transcriptional response of a whole genome to a particular event or environmental insult, giving an overall picture that was unthinkable before the advent of large scale studies. Information on entire gene regulatory networks were made available. Several studies examined the global gene expression profile of IVP embryos compared with their in vivo counterparts (McHughes et al., 2009; Mohan et al., 2004; Smith et al., 2005, 2009,). The observation of global gene expression profiles made the burden of a non-physiological environment on the early embryo transcriptome even clearer (Ecker et al., 2004.; Wrenzycki et al., 2001).

A culture-induced change in the transcriptome was observed not only between in vivo or in vitro produced embryos, but also between embryos produced in different in vitro systems. The specific composition of culture media was indeed seen to have profound effects on the relative abundance of gene transcripts in the embryo that, in turn, can have serious implications for the normality of the blastocyst (Corcoran et al., 2007; Lonergan et al., 2003a, 2006; Rizos et al., 2002a, 2003; Walker et al., 2000; Wrenzycki et al., 1998b; Wrenzycki et al., 1999; Wrenzycki et al., 2005). Even subtle changes were seen to alter the patterns of gene expression in pre-implantation embryos, such as the concentration of a single constituent (NaCl) in the culture medium (Ho et al., 1994), or the culture under suboptimal conditions for as little as 1 day (Lonergan et al., 2003a).

Detailed gene expression studies on the effect of culture media during development of the human preimplantation embryo are still missing. A paucity of material and obvious ethical restrictions make such studies difficult to undertake. It seems likely, however, that patterns of gene expression are culture-dependent also in human (Summers & Biggers, 2003). This point is of particular concern when considering the recent proliferation in media for the extended culture of human preimplantation embryos. A recent microarray analysis compared the relative transcript abundance values for blastocysts produced in ten in vitro systems, differing primarily in culture medium formulation (Côté et al., 2011). A panel of novel uncharacterized transcripts were variably expressed depending on the medium in which the blastocysts were produced. Hierarchical clustering of microarray data indicated that the closest treatment to the in vivo reference produced also one of the best blastocyst yields. Notably, the differences in transcript abundance were affected by the conditions of oocyte maturation as well.

There is considerable opportunity for the disruption of gene activity when embryos are removed from their natural environment and manipulated in vitro. Several variables during in vitro culture were seen to affect the success rate and the quality of the developing embryos. Embryo density during in vitro, for instance, significantly affected the expression of stress-related genes (de Oliveira et al., 2005), the developmental competence to blastocyst stage, as well as the gene expression patterns on a large-scale (Hoelker et al., 2009).

Evidence from studies utilizing the sheep oviduct for the post-fertilization culture of in vitro derived zygotes (Enright et al., 2000; Rizos et al., 2002a, 2002b) indicated that the period of culture after fertilization is the key part of the process responsible for suboptimal embryo quality. In vivo culture (in the ewe oviduct) of in vitro produced bovine zygotes markedly increases the quality of the resulting blastocysts, in terms of cryotolerance, to a level similar to embryos produced entirely in vivo (Enright et al., 2000; Rizos et al., 2002a, 2002b). At the transcript level, such in vivo cultured embryos showed gene expression patterns similar to true in vivo embryos (Lazzari et al., 2002; Lonergan et al., 2003a, 2003b). Similarly, the in vitro or in vivo post-fertilization environment affected the gene expression patterns of ovine embryos produced by IVM and IVF of oocytes deriving from prepubertal (Bebbere et al., 2008) and adult donors (Bogliolo et al., 2009).

While efforts are being spent to improve the efficiency of existing reproductive biotechnologies and to develop new approaches, attention should always be paid to the effects exerted by new treatment on the nascent embryos. Among the new methods proposed to improve the efficiency of in vitro embryo production systems, the exposure to sub-lethal hydrostatic pressure (HP) treatment is emerging as an approach to improve the general resistance of gametes and embryos to suboptimal conditions. While treatment with HP was seen to improve the quality of in vitro-produced ovine blastocysts by increasing their cell number and reducing the proportion of nuclear picnosis, it was also seen to alter the expression status of the blastocysts (Bogliolo et al., 2011). Whereas the change in mRNA content may give the HP exposed blastocysts a temporary higher gear, the effect on a longer term should be examined.

The observation of altered gene expression patterns in in vitro manipulated embryos with increased developmental competence raises a point on the interpretation of gene expression profiles during PED. The numerous studies that evaluated the impact of in vitro environment have mostly compared the treatment to in vivo produced embryos, which are considered to be the gold standard of quality. However, it is unlikely that embryos produced in an artificial system exhibit the same profiles as the ones that have been grown in vivo, especially because culture systems do not perfectly mimic the in vivo conditions. As such, some perturbations in the gene expression profiles should be considered normal. The question then is rather to define to what extent these perturbations are acceptable, not compromising embryonic viability or leading to deleterious long-term effects (Seli et al., 2010). Studies should be addressed to clarify the characteristics of developmental competence for an embryo cultured in vitro: is the "best" embryo the one offering the largest plasticity level and thus being able to adapt and cope with more intense environmental insults? Or is it the one that more resembles the embryo developed in vivo, maintaining its characteristics despite a non-physiological environment?

It is expected that, as it is the case in all living cells, adaptation can be stretched to a certain limit, beyond which irreversible damage will occur. The definition of embryonic competence should therefore include the level of plasticity and should be seen as an interval of acceptance rather than a clearly defined threshold value.

6. The effects of ART on genomic imprinting

While some patterns of gene expression observed as a consequence of in vitro environment seem to be compatible with a proper development of the embryo, other alterations in the embryo transcriptome consistently result in reduced quality associated with fetal and neonatal abnormalities. A substantial amount of evidence demonstrates that the culture conditions to which the embryo is exposed may perturb the epigenetic status of the embryo genome, with potentially important long-term consequences. Although linking the variations in gene expression with the observed phenotypes has been extremely challenging, it is now generally accepted that assisted reproductive technologies are associated with genomic imprinting disorders.

In mammals, genomic imprinting is an epigenetic process by which certain genes are expressed in a parent-of-origin-specific manner. It involves methylation and histone modifications in order to achieve monoallelic gene expression without altering the genetic sequence. These epigenetic marks are established in the germline, rearranged during embryonic reprogramming, and then maintained throughout all somatic cells of an organism. During PED, reprogramming involves extensive epigenetic modifications of the differentiated gamete nuclei by the ooplasm that transforms them to a totipotent embryonic nucleus. The changes in the embryo epigenome regulates the transition from maternal to embryonic control of transcription. A correct epigenetic reprogramming is needed for totipotency, correct initiation of embryonic gene expression, early lineage development, and is essential for a proper establishment of genomic imprinting in the new embryo.

Germ cell development and early embryogenesis are crucial windows in the erasure, acquisition and maintenance of genomic imprints. ART include isolation, handling and culture of gametes and early embryos at times when imprinted genes are likely to be particularly vulnerable to external influences. It is therefore predictable that in vitro manipulation during these early phases influences the epigenetic marking of the embryonic genome, and consequently its gene expression.

In recent years, concern has grown on the occurrence of disorders linked to imprinting problems in ART conceived children. Several epidemiologic studies have reported an increased frequency of imprinting defects in association with ART application (Arnaud & Feil, 2005; De Rycke et al., 2002; Owen & Segars 2009; Powell, 2003; Scarano et al., 2005; Stromberg et al., 2002; Thompson et al., 2002). Being involved in the etiology of severe developmental disorders (Arnaud & Feil, 2005; Scarano et al., 2005), such as Beckwith-Wiedemann (BWS) and Angelman Syndrome (AS), disruption of imprinting has raised particular alarm. Studies reported that the risk of AS may be increased by the use of ICSI (Cox et al., 2002; Orstavik et al., 2003), and that ART results in a three-to-six-fold-increase in the incidence of the normally rare BWS (DeBaun et al., 2003; Gicquel et al., 2003, Maher et al., 2003).

Abundant evidence on the connection between ART and altered expression of imprinted genes originates from animal models: studies performed in the mouse, sheep, and bovine species showed that the epigenetic and genetic programming of the embryo may be severely affected by in vitro environment (Lonergan et al., 2003a; Khosla et al., 2001; Young et al., 2001). Association between in vitro embryo production and disrupted imprinting resulted in a variety of abnormal phenotypes, early embryonic losses, and perinatal deaths in several mammalian species (de Sousa et al., 2001; Yang et al., 2005; Young et al., 2001; Wrenzycki & Niemann, 2003). Faulty nuclear reprogramming due to artificial manipulation is considered the primary cause of the reported defects.

In vitro culture was seen to cause abnormal epigenetic modifications and subsequent deregulation of several imprinted genes, many of which are involved in the control of pre- and postnatal growth (Walker et al., 2000). Others play important roles in regulating resource acquisition of the embryo and fetus (Isles and Wilkinson, 2000), and therefore it has been proposed that, in mammals, imprinting co-evolved with the placenta.

In ruminants, a faulty imprinting is linked to early embryonic losses, perinatal deaths, and a variety of pathological symptoms that are summarized under the term "large offspring syndrome" (LOS) (Yang et al., 2005; Young et al., 2001). Being among the best described adverse impacts of IVP, LOS comprise a series of abnormal phenotypes, such as increased gestational duration and birthweight, abnormal physiology, organ, placenta and skeletal development (McEvoy et al., 2000; Sinclair et al., 1999). It is associated with imprinting disruption (McEvoy et al., 2000; Sinclair et al., 1999; Young et al., 1998) and seems to result from the exposure of in vitro produced embryos to fetal calf serum (Farin et al., 2001; Sinclair et al., 1999, 2000). Although most pronounced in cloned embryos, LOS was reported following other types of ART, including IVF (de Sousa et al., 2001; Tilghman, 1999; Yang et al., 2005). Studies on LOS in sheep have identified altered expression level of the IGF2R imprinted gene, due to epigenetic changes (Young et al., 2001). Similar overgrowth problems seen in mice and humans are caused by errors in Igf2 and H19 imprinted genes (Eggenschwiler et al., 1997), suggesting that several genes responsible for fetal growth and development could be involved in LOS.

Notably, specific characteristics of ART-associated LOS in ruminants resemble the clinical phenotypes due to imprinting disruptions typically observed in human, such as BWS and AS (Arnaud & Feil, 2005; Scarano et al., 2005).

In rodents, studies on the preimplantation embryo suggested that particular in vitro culture conditions can alter the transcription pattern of imprinted genes and produce long-term neuro-developmental and behavioral disorders (Doherty et al., 2000; Ecker et al., 2004; Fernandez-Gonzalez et al., 2004; Humpherys et al., 2001; Mann et al., 2004; Sjoblom et al., 2005; Toppings et al., 2008). In particular, inclusion of serum in culture media was seen to alter the expression of imprinted genes and reduce the developmental potential after embryo transfer (Khosla et al., 2001). A microarray-based assessment of genomic methylation showed evidence of generalized hypermethylation, as well as greater locus-to-locus variability, in in vitro murine embryos when compared with in vivo control (Wright et al., 2011).

The alterations seen in mice, sheep and cattle in consequence of the application of ART procedures are probably relevant to most eutherian mammals, including humans. They may result from embryo exposure to suboptimal in vitro culture environments, which are incapable to supply the right signaling cues, and can lead to the deregulation of genes and aberrant epigenetic modifications (Fernandez-Gonzales et al., 2007). The sub-acute nature of some of these disruptions allows them to remain undetected in the short term, so that blastocyst production can often be achieved despite the detrimental environmental effects. However, undesirable postnatal phenotypic consequences may arise during the future development of the fetus or of the offspring, due to alteration of long-term gene expression programs (Gluckman & Hanson, 2004).

7. Conclusion

Epidemiological studies on ART conceived children and molecular analysis in several mammals yield yet contrasting results. The incomplete picture on the safety of ART demands for further studies on the basic biology of fertilization and pre-implantation development. Only a deeper understanding of the cellular and molecular mechanisms ruling life early phases will enable a proper evaluation of the severity of ART impact.

The knowledge on the regulation of gene expression is continuously advancing, unveiling a process that involves a wide range of molecules and mechanisms, and is conspicuously more complex than expected. Several classes of non coding RNAs (i.e. long non coding RNAs and microRNAs) are being recognized as crucial for the control of the transcriptome activity. Most probably, the advances in this field will transform our current concept of developmental competence and plasticity and will renovate the ideas to improve the technologies and their safety.

8. Acknowledgments

D. Bebbere was the recipient of a fellowship by Regione Autonoma della Sardegna (PO Sardegna FSE 2007-2013; L.R.7/2007).

9. References

Allen, V.M.; Wilson, R.D. & Cheung A. (2006). Pregnancy outcomes after assisted reproductive technology. *J Obstet Gynaecol Can*; 28, 220–33.

Andersen, A.N.; Carlsen, E. & Loft, A. (2008). Trends in the use of intracytoplasmatic sperm injection marked variability between countries. *Human Reproduction Update,* 14, 593–604.

Arnaud, P. & Feil, R. (2005). Epigenetic deregulation of genomic imprinting in human disorders and following assisted reproduction. *Birth Defects Res C Embryo Today*, 75, 81–97.

Barker D.J. (1997). Maternal nutrition, fetal nutrition, and disease in later life. *Nutrition,* 13, 807-13.

Basso, O. & Baird, D.D. (2003). Infertility and preterm delivery, birth weight, and Caesarean section: a study within the Danish National Birth Cohort. *Hum Reprod,* 18, 2478–84.

Bebbere, D.; Bogliolo, L., Ariu, F., Fois, S., Leoni, G.G., Tore, S., Succu, S., Berlinguer, F., Naitana, S. & Ledda, S. (2008). Expression pattern of zygote arrest 1 (ZAR1), maternal antigen that embryo requires (MATER), growth differentiation factor 9 (GDF9) and bone morphogenetic protein 15 (BMP15) genes in ovine oocytes and in vitro-produced preimplantation embryos. *Reprod Fertil Dev,* 20, 908-15.

Bebbere, D.; Bogliolo, L., Fois, S., Ariu, F., Leoni, G.G., Berlinguer, F., Naitana, S.& Ledda, S. (2008) In vitro or in vivo post-fertilization embryo culture affects the gene expression patterns of ovine prepubertal embryos. *Proceeding of the 1st GEMINI MEETING, Volos, Greece,* 9th-12th October 2008, page 17.

Bensaude, O. & Morange, M. (1983). Spontaneous high expression of heat-shock proteins in mouse embryonal carcinoma cells and ectoderm from day 8 mouse embryo. *EMBO J,* 2, 173-7.

Bergh, T.; Ericson, A., Hillensjö, T., Nygren, K.G. & Wennerholm, U.B. (1997). Deliveries and children born after in vitro fertilization in Sweden 1982–95: a retrospective cohort study. *Lancet*, 354, 1579–85.

Bettegowda, A.; Yao, J., Sen, A., , Li, Q., Lee, K.B., Kobayashi, Y., Patel, O.V., Coussens, P.M., Ireland, J.J. & Smith, G.W. (2007). JY-1, an oocyte-specific gene, regulates granulosa cell function and early embryonic development in cattle. *Proc Natl Acad Sci USA*, 104, 17602-7.

Bogliolo, L.; Bebbere, D., Ariu, F., Pintus, E., Strina, A., Succu, S. & Ledda, S. (2009). In vitro or in vivo post-fertilization embryo culture affects the gene expression patterns of ovine embryos. *Proceeding of the 2nd General Meeting of GEMINI*, Sardinia, Italy, 1st - 3rd October, page 51.

Bogliolo, L.; Ariu, F., Leoni, G., Uccheddu, S. & Bebbere, D. (2011). High hydrostatic pressure treatment improves the quality of in vitro-produced ovine blastocysts. *Reprod Fertil Dev*, 23, 809-17.

Bonduelle, M.; Legein, J., Buysse, A., Van Assche, E., Wisanto, A., Devroey, P., Van Steirteghem, A.C. & Liebaers, I. (1996). Prospective follow-up study of 423 children born after intracytoplasmic sperm injection. *Hum Reprod.*, 11, 1558-64.

Camous, S.; Kopecný, V. & Fléchon, J.E. (1986). Autoradiographic detection of the earliest stage of [3H]-uridine incorporation into the cow embryo. *Biol Cell*, 58, 195-200.

Christians, E.; Campion, E., Thompson, E.M. & Renard, J.P. (1995). Expression of the HSP 70.1 gene, a landmark of early zygotic activity in the mouse embryo, is restricted to the first burst of transcription. *Development*, 121, 113-22.

Corcoran, D.; Rizos, D., Fair, T., Evans, A.C. & Lonergan, P. (2007). Temporal expression of transcripts related to embryo quality in bovine embryos cultured from the two-cell to blastocyst stage in vitro or in vivo. *Mol Reprod Dev*, 74, 972-7.

Côté, I.; Vigneault, C., Laflamme, I., Laquerre, J., Fournier, E., Gilbert, I., Scantland, S., Gagné, D., Blondin, P. & Robert C. (2011). Comprehensive cross production system assessment of the impact of in vitro microenvironment on the expression of messengers and long non-coding RNAs in the bovine blastocyst. *Reproduction*, 142, 99-112.

Cox, G.F.; Burger, J., Lip, V., Mau, U.A., Sperling, K., Wu, B.L. & Horsthemke, B. (2002). Intracytoplasmic sperm injection may increase the risk of imprinting defects. *Am. J. Hum. Genet.*, 71, 162–164.

Cui, X.S. & Kim, N.H. (2007). Maternally derived transcripts: identification and characterisation during oocyte maturation and early cleavage. *Reprod Fertil Dev.*, 19, 25-34.

Dade, S.; Callebaut, I., Paillisson, A., Bontoux, M., Dalbies-Tran, R., & Monget, P. (2004). In silico identification and structural features of six new genes similar to MATER specifically expressed in the oocyte. *Biochem. Biophys. Res. Commun.* 324, 547–553.

de Oliveira A.T.; Lopes, R.F. & Rodrigues, J.L. (2005). Gene expression and developmental competence of bovine embryos produced in vitro under varying embryo density conditions. *Theriogenology*, 64, 1559–1572.

De Rycke, M.; Liebaers, I. & Van Steirteghem, A. (2002). Epigenetic risks related to assisted reproductive technologies: risk analysis and epigenetic inheritance. *Hum Reprod* 17, 2487–2494.

De Sousa P.A.; King, T., Harkness, L., Young, L.E., Walker, S.K. & Wilmut, I. (2001). Evaluation of gestational deficiencies in cloned sheep fetuses and placentae. *Biol Reprod.*, 65, 23-30.

Dean, J. (2002). Oocyte-specific genes regulate follicle formation, fertility and early mouse development. *J Reprod Immunol,* 53, 171–180.

DeBaun, M.R.; Niemitz, E.L. & Feinberg, A.P. (2003) Association of in vitro fertilization with Beckwith–Wiedemann syndrome and epigenetic alterations of LIT1 and H19. *Am. J. Hum. Genet.*, 72, 156–160.

Doherty, A.S.; Mann, M.R., Tremblay, K.D., Bartolomei, M.S. & Schultz, R.M. (2000). Differential effects of culture on imprinted H19 expression in the preimplantation mouse embryo. *Biol. Reprod.*, 62, 1526.

Draper, E.S.; Kurinczuk, J.J., Abrams, K.R. & Clarke, M. (1999). Assessment of separate contributions to perinatal mortality of infertility history and treatment: a case-control analysis. *Lancet*, 353, 1746–49.

Ecker, D.J.; Stein, P., Xu, Z., Williams, C.J., Kopf, G.S., Bilker, W.B., Abel, T. & Schultz, R.M. (2004). Long-term effects of culture of preimplantation mouse embryos on behavior. *Proc Natl Acad Sci USA*, 101, 1595–600.

Eggenschwiler, J.; Ludwig, T., Fisher, P., Leighton, P.A., Tilghman, S.M. & Efstratiadis, A. (1997). Mouse mutant embryos overexpressing IGF-II exhibit phenotypic features of the Beckwith-Wiedemann and Simpson-Golabi-Behmel syndromes. *Genes Dev.*, 11, 3128-42.

Enright, B.P.; Lonergan, P., Dinnyes, A., Fair, T., Ward, F.A., Yang, X. & Boland, M.P. (2000). Culture of in vitro produced bovine zygotes in vitro vs in vivo: implications for early embryo development and quality. *Theriogenology;* 54, 659-73.

Farin, P.W.; Crosier, A.E. & Farin, C.E. (2001). Influence of in vitro systems on embryo survival and fetal development in cattle. *Theriogenology*, 55, 151-70.

Fernández-Gonzalez, R.; Moreira, P., Bilbao, A., Jiménez, A., Pérez-Crespo, M., Ramírez, M.A., Rodríguez De Fonseca, F., Pintado, B. & Gutiérrez-Adán, A. (2004). Long-term effect of in vitro culture of mouse embryos with serum on mRNA expression of imprinting genes, development, and behavior. *Proc Natl Acad Sci USA*, 101, 5880-5.

Fernández-Gonzalez, R.; Ramirez, M.A., Bilbao, A., De Fonseca, F.R. & Gutiérrez-Adán, A. (2007). Suboptimal in vitro culture conditions: an epigenetic origin of long-term health effects. *Mol Reprod Dev.*, 74, 1149-56.

Foote RH. (1982). Cryopreservation of spermatozoa and artificial insemination: past, present and future. *J Androl*, 3, 85–100.

Friedler, S.; Mashiach, S. & Laufer, N. (1992). Births in Israel resulting from in-vitro fertilization/embryo transfer, 1982-1989: National registry of the Israeli association for fertility research *Human Reproduction* 7:8 (1159-1163).

Ghazi, H.A.; Spielberger, C. & Kallen B. (1991). Delivery outcome after infertility: a registry study. *Fertil Steril.*, 55, 726–32.

Gicquel, C.; Gaston, V., Mandelbaum, J., Siffro, J-P., Flahault, A. & Le Bouc, Y. (2003). In vitro fertilization may increase the risk of Beckwith–Widemann syndrome related to abnormal imprinting of the KCNQ1OT gene. *Am. J. Hum. Genet.*, 72, 1338–1341.

Gilbert, S.F. *Developmental biology,* 6th ed. Sunderland MA: Sinauer Associates; 2000.

Gluckman, P.D. & Hanso,n M.A. (2004). Developmental origins of disease paradigm: a mechanistic and evolutionary perspective. *Pediatr Res.*, 56, 311-7.

Gosden, R.G.; Baird, D.T., Wade, J.C. & Webb, R. (1994). Restoration of fertility to oophorectomized sheep by ovarian autografts stored at -196 degrees C. *Hum Reprod.*, 9, 597-603.

Grace, K.S. & Sinclair, K.D. (2009). Assisted Reproductive Technology, Epigenetics, and Long-Term Health: A Developmental Time Bomb Still Ticking. *Semin Reprod Med,* 27, 409–416.

Greve, T.; Callesen, H., Hyttel, P. & Avery, B. (1995). *From oocyte to calf In vivo and in vitro.* In: Greppi GF and Enne G (eds) Animal Production and Biotechnology. Biofutur, Paris, 1995, 71-97.

Gutiérrez-Adán, A.; Rizo,s D., Fair, T., Moreira, P.N., Pintado, B., de la Fuente, J., Boland, M.P. & Lonergan, P. (2004). Effect of speed of development on mRNA expression pattern in early bovine embryos cultured in vivo or in vitro. *Mol Reprod Dev*, 68, 441-8.

Hamatani, T.; Carter, M.G., Sharov, A.A. & Ko, M.S. (2004). Dynamics of global gene expression changes during mouse preimplantation development. *Dev Cell,* 6, 117–31.

Hansen, M.; Kurinczuk, J.J., Bower, C. & Webb, S.N. (2002). The risk of major birth defects after intracytoplasmic sperm injection and in vitro fertilization. *N Engl J Med.,* 356, 725-730.

Henriksen, T.B.; Baird, D.D., Olsen, J., Hedegaard, M., Secher, N.J. & Wilcox, A.J. (1997). Time to pregnancy and preterm delivery. *Obstet Gynecol,* 89, 594–99.

Ho, Y.; Doherty, A.S. & Schultz, R.M. (1994). Mouse preimplantation embryo development in vitro: effect of sodium concentration in culture media on RNA synthesis and accumulation and gene expression. *Mol Reprod Dev.*, 38, 131-41.

Hoelker, M.; Rings, F., Lund, Q., Ghanem, N., Phatsara, C., Griese, J., Schellander, K. & Tesfaye, D. (2009). Effect of the microenvironment and embryo density on developmental characteristics and gene expression profile of bovine preimplantative embryos cultured in vitro. *Reproduction.*, 137, 415-25.

Humpherys, D.; Eggan, K., Akutsu, H., Hochedlinger, K., Rideout, W.M. 3rd, Biniszkiewicz, D., Yanagimachi, R. & Jaenisch, R. (2001). Epigenetic instability in ES cells and cloned mice. *Science*, 293, 95–7.

Isles, A.R. & Wilkinson, L.S. (2000). Imprinted genes, cognition and behaviour. *Trends Cogn Sci.*, 4, 309-318.

Jackson, R.A.; Gibson, K.A., Wu, Y.W. & Croughan, M.S. (2004). Perinatal outcomes in singletons following in vitro fertilization: a meta-analysis. *Obstet Gynecol*, 103, 551–63.

Khosla, S.; Dean, W., Reik, W. & Feil, R. (2001). Culture of pre implantation embryos and its long-term eff ects on gene expression and phenotype. *Hum Reprod Update*, 7, 419–27.

Knijn, H.M.; Wrenzycki, C., Hendriksen, P.J., Vos, P.L., Zeinstra, E.C., van der Weijden, G.C., Niemann, H. & Dieleman, S.J. (2005). In vitro and in vivo culture effects on mRNA expression of genes involved in metabolism and apoptosis in bovine embryos. *Reprod Fertil Dev.*, 17, 775-84.

Kopecny, V. (1989). High-resolution autoradiographic studies of comparative nucleologenesis and genome reactivation during early embryogenesis in pig, man and cattle. *Reprod Nutr Dev*, 29, 589–600.

Kurinczuk, J.J. & Bower, C. (1997). Birth defects in infants conceived by intracytoplasmic sperm injection: an alternative interpretation. *Br Med J* 315, 1260-1265.

Lazzari, G.; Wrenzycki, C., Herrmann, D., Duchi, R., Kruip, T., Niemann, H. & Galli, C. (2002). Cellular and molecular deviations in bovine in vitro-produced embryos are related to the large offspring syndrome. Biol Reprod., 67, 767-75.

Leibo, S.P. & Loskutoff, N.M. (1993). Cryobiology of in vitro-derived bovine embryos. *Theriogenology*, 43, 81-9.

Lonergan, P.; Rizos, D., Gutiérrez-Adán, A., Fair, T. & Boland, M.P. (2003a). Effect of culture environment on embryo quality and gene expression - experience from animal studies. *Reprod Biomed Online*, 7, 657-63.

Lonergan, P.; Rizos, D., Gutierrez-Adan, A., Fair, T. & Boland, M.P. (2003b). Oocyte and embryo quality: effect of origin, culture conditions and gene expression patterns. *Reprod Domest Anim*, 38, 259-67.

Lonergan, P.; Fair, T., Corcoran, D., & Evans, A.C. (2006). Effect of culture environment on gene expression and developmental characteristics in IVF-derived embryos. *Theriogenology*, 65, 137-52.

Maher, E.R.; Brueton, L.A., Bowdin, S.C., Luharia, A., Cooper, W., Cole, T.R., Macdonald, F., Sampson, J.R., Barratt, C.L., Reik, W. & Hawkins, M.M. (2003). Beckwith-Wiedemann syndrome and assisted reproduction technology (ART). *J. Med. Genet.*, 40, 62–64.

Mann, M.R.; Lee, S.S., Doherty, A.S., Verona, R.I., Nolen, L.D., Schultz, R.M. & Bartolomei, M.S. (2004). Selective loss of imprinting in the placenta following preimplantation development in culture. *Development*, 131, 3727–3735.

McDonald, S.D.; Murphy, K., Beyene, J. & Ohlsson, A. (2005). Perinatal outcome of singleton pregnancies achieved by in vitro fertilization: a systematic review and meta-analysis. *J Obstet Gynaecol Can*, 27, 449–59.

McDonald, S.D.; Han, Z., Mulla, S., Murphy, K.E., Beyene, J. & Ohlsson, A. (2009). Knowledge Synthesis Group. Preterm birth and low birth weight among in vitro fertilization singletons: a systematic review and meta-analyses. *Eur J Obstet Gynecol Reprod Biol.*, 146, 138-48.

McEvoy, T.G.; Sinclair, K.D., Young, L.E., Wilmut, I. & Robinson, J.J. (2000). Large offspring syndrome and other consequences of ruminant embryo culture in vitro: relevance to blastocyst culture in human ART. *Hum Fertil (Camb).*, 3, 238-246.

McEvoy, T.G.; Robinson, J.J. & Sinclair, K.D. (2001). Developmental consequences of embryo and cell manipulation in mice and farm animals. *Reproduction*, 122, 507–18.

McGovern PG, Llorens AJ, Skurnick JH, Weiss G, Goldsmith LT. Increased risk of preterm birth in singleton pregnancies resulting from in vitro fertilization-embryo transfer or gamete intrafallopian transfer: a meta-analysis. Fertil Steril 2004; 82: 1514–20.

McHughes, C.E.; Springer, G.K., Spate, L.D., Li, R., Woods, R., Green, M.P., Korte, S.W., Murphy, C.N., Green, J.A. & Prather, R.S. (2009). Identification and quantification of differentially represented transcripts in in vitro and in vivo derived preimplantation bovine embryos. *Molecular Reproduction and Development*, 76, 48–60.

Misirlioglu, M.; Page, G.P., Sagirkaya, H., Kaya, A., Parrish, J.J., First, N.L. & Memili, E. (2006). Dynamics of global transcriptome in bovine matured oocytes and preimplantation embryos. *Proc Natl Acad Sci USA*, 103, 18905–10.

Mohan, M.; Hurst, A.G. & Malayer, J.R. (2004). Global gene expression analysis comparing bovine blastocysts flushed on day 7 or produced in vitro. *Molecular Reproduction and Development*, 68, 288–298.

Niemann, H. (1995). Advances in cryopreservation of bovine oocytes and embryos derived in vitro and in vivo. In: *Reproduction and Animal Breeding. Advances and Strategy* (Eds G. Enne, G.F.. Greppi and A. Lauria), Elsevier Biofutur, 117-128.

Niemann, H. & Wrenzycki, C. (2000). Alterations of expression of developmentally important genes in preimplantation bovine embryos by in vitro culture conditions: implications for subsequent development. *Theriogenology*, 53, 21-34.

Nyholt de Prada, J.K.; Kellam, L.D., Patel, B.G., Latham, K.E. & Vandevoort, C.A. (2010). Growth hormone and gene expression of in vitro-matured rhesus macaque oocytes. *Mol Reprod Dev*, 77, 353–62.

Oh, B.; Hwang, S., McLaughlin, J., Solter, D. & Knowles, B.B. (2000). Timely translation during the mouse oocyte-to-embryo transition. *Development*, 127, 3795-803.

Orstavik, K.H.; Eiklid, K., van der Hagen, C.B., Spetalen, S., Kierulf, K., Skjeldal, O. and Buiting, K. (2003). Another case of imprinting defect in a girl with Angelman syndrome who was conceived by intracytoplasmic semen injection. *Am. J. Hum. Genet.*, 42, 218–219.

Owen, C.M. & Segars, J.H. Jr. (2009). Imprinting disorders and assisted reproductive technology. *Semin Reprod Med.*, 27, 417-28.

Palermo, G.; Joris, H., Devroey, P. & Van Steirteghem, A.C. (1992). Pregnancies after intracytoplasmic injection of single spermatozoon into an oocyte. *Lancet*, 340, 17–18.

Pangas, S.A. & Rajkovic, A. (2006). Transcriptional regulation of early oogenesis: in search of masters. *Human Reproduction Update*, 12, 65–76.

Pennetier, S.; Uzbekova, S., Perreau, C. Papillier, P., Mermillod, P., Dalbiès-Tran, R. (2004). Spatio-Temporal Expression of the Germ Cell Marker Genes *MATER, ZAR1, GDF9, BMP15,* and *VASA* in Adult Bovine Tissues, Oocytes, and Preimplantation Embryos. *Biol Reprod*, 71, 1359–1366.

Pennetier, S., Perreau, C., Uzbekova, S., Thélie, A., Delaleu, B., Mermillod, P., Dalbiès-Tran, R. (2006). MATER protein expression and intracellular localization throughout folliculogenesis and preimplantation embryo development in the bovine. *BMC Dev Biol.*, 6, 26.

Pikó, L. & Clegg, K.B. (1982). Quantitative changes in total RNA, total poly(A), and ribosomes in early mouse embryos. *Dev Biol.*, 89, 362-78.

Polge. C.; Smith, A.U. & Parkes, A.S. (1949). Revival of spermatozoa after vitrification and dehydration at low temperatures. *Nature*, 164, 666.

Powell, K. (2003). Fertility treatments: seeds of doubt. *Nature* 422, 656–658.

Rajkovic, A. & Matzuk, M. M. (2002). Functional analysis of oocyte expressed genes using transgenic models. *Mol. Cell. Endocrinol.*, 187, 5–9.

Richter, J.D. (1999). Cytoplasmic polyadenylation in development and beyond. *Microbiol Mol Biol Rev*, 63, 446-56.

Rizos, D.; Lonergan, P., Boland, M.P., Arroyo-Garcia, R., Pintado, B., de la Fuente, J. & Gutierrez-Adan, A. (2002a). Analysis of differential messenger RNA expression between bovine blastocysts produced in different culture systems: Implications for blastocyst quality. *Biol Reprod*, 66, 589–595.

Rizos, D.; Ward, F., Duffy, P., Boland, M.P. & Lonergan, P. (2002b). Consequences of bovine oocyte maturation, fertilization or early embryo development in vitro versus in vivo: Implications for blastocyst yield and blastocyst quality. *Mol Reprod Dev*, 61, 234–248.

Rizos, D.; Gutierrez-Adan, A., Perez-Garnelo, S., De La Fuente, J., Boland, M.P. & Lonergan, P. (2003). Bovine embryo culture in the presence or absence of serum: Implications for blastocyst development, cryotolerance, and messenger RNA expression. *Biol Reprod*. 68, 236–243.

Romundstad, L.B.; Romundstad, P.R., Sunde, A., von Düring, V., Skjaerven, R., Gunnell, D. & Vatten, L.J. (2008). Effects of technology or maternal factors on perinatal outcome after assisted fertilisation: a population-based cohort study. *Lancet*, 372, 737-43.

Saunders, D.M. & Lancaster P.A. (1989). The wider perinatal significance of the Australian in vitro fertilization data collection program. *Am J Perinatol.*, 6, 252-7.

Scarano, M.I.; Strazzullo, M., Matarazzo, M.R. & D'Esposito, M. (2005). DNA methylation 40 years later: its role in human health and disease. *J Cell Physio,l* 204, 21–35.

Schieve, L.A.; Meikle, S.F., Ferre, C., Peterson, H.B., Jeng, G. & Wilcox, L.S. (2002). Low and very low birth weight in infants conceived with use of assisted reproductive technology. *N. Engl. J. Med.*, 346, 731–737.

Schultz, R.M. (1993). Regulation of zygotic gene activation in the mouse. *Bioessays*, 15, 531–8.

Seli, E.; Robert, C. & Sirard, M.A. (2010). OMICS in assisted reproduction: possibilities and pitfalls. *Molecular Human Reproduction*, 16, 513–530.

Seydoux, G. (1996). Mechanisms of translational control in early development. *Curr Opin Genet Dev*, 6, 555-61.

Sinclair, K.D.; McEvoy, T.G., Maxfield, E.K., Maltin, C.A., Young, L.E., Wilmut, I., Broadbent, P.J., Robinson, J.J. (1999). Aberrant fetal growth and development after in vitro culture of sheep zygotes. *J Reprod Fertil.*, 116, 177-86.

Sinclair, K.D.; Young, L.E., Wilmut, I. & McEvoy, T.G. (2000). In-utero overgrowth in ruminants following embryo culture: lessons from mice and a warning to men. *Hum Reprod.*, 15, suppl. 5, 68-86.

Sjöblom, C., Roberts, C.T., Wikland, M. & Robertson, S.A. (2005). Granulocyte-macrophage colony-stimulating factor alleviates adverse consequences of embryo culture on fetal growth trajectory and placental morphogenesis. *Endocrinology.*, 146, 2142-53.

Smith, S.L.; Everts, R.E., Tian, X.C., Du, F., Sung, L.Y., Rodriguez-Zas, S.L., Jeong, B.S., Renard, J.P., Lewin, H.A. & Yang, X. (2005). Global gene expression profiles reveal significant nuclear reprogramming by the blastocyst stage after cloning. *Proc Natl Acad Sci USA*, 102, 17582-7.

Smith, S.L.; Everts, R.E., Sung, L.Y., Du, F., Page, R.L., Henderson, B., Rodriguez-Zas, S.L., Nedambale, T.L., Renard, J.P., Lewin, H.A., Yang, X. & Tian, X.C. (2009). Gene expression profiling of single bovine embryos uncovers significant effects of in vitro maturation, fertilization and culture. *Mol Reprod Dev.*, 76, 38-47. Erratum in: *Mol Reprod Dev.*, 76, 523.

Solter, D. (2002). Cloning v. clowning. *Genes Dev*, 16, 1163-6.

Steptoe, P.C. & Edwards, R.G. (1978). Birth after the reimplantation of a human embryo. *Lancet* 2, 366.

Stromberg, B.; Dahlquist, G., Ericson, A., Finnstrom, O., Koster, M. & Stjernqvist, K. (2002). Neurological sequelae in children born after in-vitro fertilisation: a population-based study. *Lancet*, 359, 461–465.

Summers, M.C. & Biggers, J.D. (2003). Chemically defined media and the culture of mammalian preimplantation embryos: Historical perspective and current issues. *Hum Reprod Update*, 9, 557–82.

Sutcliff, A.G. & Ludwig, M. (2007). Outcome of assisted reproduction. *Lancet*, 370, 351–59.

Telford, N.A.; Watson, A.J. & Schultz, G.A. (1990). Transition from maternal to embryonic control in early mammalian development a comparison of several species. *Mol Reprod Dev*, 26, 90–100.

Tesfaye, D.; Ponsuksili, S., Wimmers, K., Gilles, M. & Schellander, K. (2004). A comparative expression analysis of gene transcripts in post-fertilization developmental stages of bovine embryos produced in vitro or in vivo. *Reprod Domest Anim.*, 39, 396-404.

Thelie, A.; Papillier, P., Pennetier, S., Perreau, C., Traverso, J. M., Uzbekova, S., Mermillod, P., Joly, C., Humblot, P., & Dalbies-Tran, R. (2007). Differential regulation of abundance and deadenylation of maternal transcripts during bovine oocyte maturation in vitro and in vivo. *BMC Dev. Biol.*, 7, 125.

Thompson, J.G.; Kind, K.L., Roberts, C.T., Robertson, S.A. & Robinson, J.S. (2002). Epigenetic risks related to assisted reproductive technologies: short- and long-term consequences for the health of children conceived through assisted reproduction technology: more reason for caution? *Hum Reprod.*, 17, 2783-6.

Tilghman, S.M. (1999). The sins of the fathers and mothers: genomic imprinting in mammalian development. *Cell*, 96, 185–93.

Tong, Z. B.; Bondy, C. A., Zhou, J., & Nelson, L. M. (2002). A human homologue of mouse Mater, a maternal effect gene essential for early embryonic development. *Hum. Reprod.*, 17, 903–911.

Toppings, M,; Castro, C., Mills, P.H., Reinhart, B., Schatten, G., Ahrens, E.T., Chaillet, J.R. & Trasler, J.M. (2008). Profound phenotypic variation among mice deficient in the maintenance of genomic imprints. *Hum Reprod.*, 23, 807-18.

Uechi, H.; Tsutsumi, O., Morita, Y. & Taketani, Y. (1997). Cryopreservation of mouse embryos affects later embryonic development possibly through reduced expression of the glucose transporter GLUT1. *Mol Reprod Dev.*, 48, 496-500.

Uzbekova, S.; Roy-Sabau, M., Dalbiès-Tran, R., Perreau, C., Papillier, P., Mompart, F., Thelie, A., Pennetier, S., Cognie, J., Cadoret, V., Royere, D., Monget, P. & Mermillod, P. (2006). Zygote arrest 1 gene in pig, cattle and human evidence of different transcript variants in male and female germ cells. *Reprod. Biol. Endocrinol.*, 4, 12.

Vigneault, C.; Gravel, C., Valle´e, M., McGraw, S. & Sirard, M.A. (2009a). Unveiling the bovine embryo transcriptome during the maternal-to-embryonic transition. *Reproduction*, 137, 245–257.

Vigneault, C,; McGraw, S. & Sirard, M.A. (2009b). Spatiotemporal expression of transcriptional regulators in concert with the maternal-to-embryonic transition during bovine in vitro embryogenesis. Reproduction, 137, 13–21.

Walker, S.R.; Hartwich, K.M. & Robinson, J,S. (2000). Long-term effects on offspring of exposure of oocytes and embryos to chemical and physical agents. *Hum Reprod Update*, 6, 564–577.

Williams, M.A.; Goldman, M.B., Mittendorf, R. & Monson, R.R. (1991). Subfertility and the risk of low birth weight. *Fertil Steril.*, 56, 668–71.

Wrenzycki, C.; Herrmann, D., Carnwath, J.W. & Niemann, H. (1996). Expression of the gap junction gene connexin43 (Cx43) in preimplantation bovine embryos derived in vitro or in vivo. *J Reprod Fertil*, 108, 17-24.

Wrenzycki, C.; Herrmann, D., Lemme, E., Korsawe, K., Carnwath, J.W. & Niemann, H. (1998a). Determination of the relative abundance of various developmentally important gene transcripts in bovine embryos generated in vitro or in vivo using a semi-quantitative RT-PCR assay. In: IETS Satellite Workshop Proceedings *"Embryo development in vitro: current challenges and future concepts"*, 14- 15.

Wrenzycki, C.; Herrmann, D., Carnwath, J.W. & Niemann H. (1998b). Expression of RNA from developmentally important genes in preimplantation bovine embryos produced in TCM supplemented with BSA. *J Reprod Fertil,*112, 387-398.

Wrenzycki, C.; Herrmann, D., Carnwath, J.W. & Niemann, H. (1999). Alterations in the relative abundance of gene transcripts in preimplantation bovine embryos cultured in medium supplemented with either serum or PVA. *Mol Reprod Dev,* 53, 8-18.

Wrenzycki, C.; Hermann, D., Keskintepe, L., Martins, A. Jr., Sirisathien, S., Brackett, B. & Niemann, H. (2001). Effects of basic culture and protein supplementation on mRNA expression in preimplantation bovine embryos. *Hum Reprod,* 16, 893–901.

Wrenzycki, C. & Niemann, H. (2003). Epigenetic reprogramming in early embryonic development: effects of in-vitro production and somatic nuclear transfer. *Reprod Biomed Online.*, 7, 649-56.

Wrenzycki, C.; Herrmann, D., Lucas-Hahn, A., Korsawe, K., Lemme, E. & Niemann, H. (2005). Messenger RNA expression patterns in bovine embryos derived from in vitro procedures and their implications for development. *Reprod Fertil Dev,* 17, 23-35.

Wright, K.; Brown, L., Brown, G., Casson, P. & Brown, S. (2011). Microarray assessment of methylation in individual mouse blastocyst stage embryos shows that in vitro culture may have widespread genomic effects. *Hum Reprod.*, 26, 2576-85.

Wu, X.; Viveiros, M.M., Eppig, J.J., Bai, Y., Fitzpatrick, S.L. & Matzuk, M.M. (2003). Zygote arrest 1 (Zar1) is a novel maternal-effect gene critical for the oocyte-to-embryo transition. *Nat Genet*, 33, 187–191.

Xie, D.; Chen, C.C., Ptaszek, L.M., Xiao, S., Cao, X., Fang, F., Ng, H.H., Lewin, H.A., Cowan, C. & Zhong, S. (2010). Rewirable gene regulatory networks in the preimplantation embryonic development of three mammalian species. *Genome Res,* 20, 804-15.

Yang, L.; Chavatte-Palmer, P., Kubota, C., O'neill, M., Hoagland, T., Renard, J.P., Taneja, M., Yang, X. & Tian, X.C. (2005). Expression of imprinted genes is aberrant in deceased newborn cloned calves and relatively normal in surviving adult clones. *Mol Reprod Dev*, 71, 431–8.

Young, L.E.; Sinclair, K.D. & Wilmut, I. (1998). Large offspring syndrome in cattle and sheep. *Rev Reprod.*, 3, 155-63.

Young, L.E.; Fernandes, K., McEvoy, T.G., Butterwith, S.C., Gutierrez, C.G., Carolan, C., Broadbent, P.J., Robinson, J.J., Wilmut, I. & Sinclair, K.D. (2001). Epigenetic change in IGF2R is associated with fetal overgrowth after sheep embryo culture. Nat Genet, 27, 153–4.

Zhang, M.; Ouyang, H. & Xia, G. (2009a). The signal pathway of gonadotrophins-induced mammalian oocyte meiotic resumption. *Mol Hum Reprod,* 15, 399–409.

Zhang, P.; Zucchelli, M., Bruce, S., Hambiliki, F., Stavreus-Evers, A., Levkov, L., Skottman, H., Kerkelä, E., Kere, J. & Hovatta O. (2009b). Transcriptome profiling of human pre-implantation development. *PloS one;* 4: e7844.

7

Third Millennium Assisted Reproductive Technologies: The Impact of Oocyte Vitrification

P. Boyer[1], P. Rodrigues[2], P. Tourame[1], M. Silva[2,4], M. Barata[2], J. Perez-Alzaa[3] and M. Gervoise-Boyer[1]

[1]*Service de Médecine et Biologie de la Reproduction Hôpital Saint Joseph Marseille,*
[2]*CMR British Hospital Lisboa*
[3]*Fundacion Fecundart - Universidad Nacional de Cordoba,*
[4]*Faculdade de Medicina da Universidade de Lisboa,*
[1]*France*
[3]*Argentina*
[2,4]*Portugal*

1. Introduction

IVF has been widely used since 1978 (Steptoe & Edwards, 1978) to help infertile couples conceive when nature has failed. The IVF field was improved through embryo freezing/thawing, a technique developed by A. Trounson (Trounson & Mohr, 1983). The next major innovation came with ICSI in 1992, through the work of G.P. Palermo (Palermo et al., 1992). C. Chen was the first to publish work on oocyte freezing (Chen, 1986), but results remained too unreliable for this technique to be adopted in routine ART practice. Oocyte freezing became the focus of experimental efforts when in 1999 the first birth using oocyte vitrification was reported by L. Kuleshova (Kuleshova et al., 1999). M. Kuwayama in a 2005 publication confirmed that this new procedure could be useful in clinical practice (Kuwayama et al., 2005). Within a few years his method for freezing the human oocyte has become the standard for the field. Its clinical application has been widely developed and is now routine, even if other variants have since been proposed. There have been efforts to assess the safety of the procedure (Chian et al., 2008, Noyes et al., 2009). Noteworthy is R. Chian's report on the health of 200 babies born after having been conceived with vitrified oocytes. The safety of the procedure is also supported by all the data available on the health of children born from vitrified embryos (Takahashi et al., 2005, Mukaida et al., 2009). Use of the technique has reached France (Boyer et al., 2010) with passage of a new bioethics law in the summer of 2011. From Italy we have a good overview of what takes place on a nation-wide basis once the technique has become standard practice, thanks to the yearly report of ART results published by the country's ministry of health (Relazione del Ministro della Salute, anno 2009).

Some issues are still being debated, e.g. an open versus closed system, infectious risks with Liquid Nitrogen (LN), the safety of cryoprotectants, the health of the unborn children. It is known that for oocyte vitrification to be most successful an open system is still needed, as shown recently by Paffoni and colleagues (Paffoni et al., 2011). The major concern with regard to an open system is the risk of LN-mediated transmission of infective agents. Researchers testing the safety of the closed system have shown it is possible to introduce contaminants voluntarily into a LN environment. They have suggested taking certain precautions when using an open system. To safeguard samples in the storage container, they recommend sealing the samples after cooling and prior to storage (Bielanski & Vajta, 2009). Parmegiani and colleagues (Parmegiani et al., 2010) suggest sterilizating LN by UV light. However, though safe and easy, UV sterilization is a costly procedure. The debate over the health of children born through oocyte vitrification is one that will not be resolved overnight. However, all the evidence published so far is reassuring. We should remember that when IVF, embryo freezing/thawing and ICSI were first developed, each advance was faced with similar resistance. What has changed is the success of national health authorities in imposing "precaution as a rule" as the only politically correct point of view. Most forget they would have probably banished IVF or ICSI back in the old days. Fortunately, international collaborations have produced quality studies which demonstrate that this new method is almost as safe as the slow-freezing method (Gook & Edgar, 2007, 2009, Cutting et al., 2009; Dessolle et al., 2009; Fadini et al., 2009, Nagy et al., 2009; Smith et al., 2010, Parmegiani et al., 2011). Good results for zygotes (Al-Hasani et al., 2007), day-2 or 3 embryos (Balaban et al., 2008) and embryos in blastocyst phase (Mukaida et al., 2009) have been obtained. The superiority to slow-freezing and the adaptability of fast-freezing to a closed system have also been demonstrated for embryos (VanderZwalmen et al., 2007) but these improvements will have fewer consequences for the future of ART than egg freezing. The new technique will probably render obsolete the cumbersome programmable freezers (Vajta & Nagy, 2009), but that is a mere detail compared to the other gains that can be expected. At this juncture, we must remember our debt to R. Edwards. We continue to be guided by both his brilliant work and his fearlessness and combativity in the cause of innovation, which led to international recognition and eventually the Nobel Prize. The message is clear: we must carry on his footsteps.

Cryobiology has developed steadily over several decades and along with ICSI has provided the conditions for a new clinical approach to ART practice. We are now ready to adopt oocyte vitrification in our biological and clinical procedures. The changes will lead to a more efficient and probably more humane practice.

2. Vitrification: Its importance in IVF

2.1 Increasing the number of fresh embryo transfers

The new approach allows cryopreservation of a part of the oocyte cohort, rather than creating embryos and then freezing any unused ones. Until now, because of the very short lifetime of this particular cell, the procedure required that we fertilize all mature oocytes, verify fertilization, discard all unfertilized oocytes and freeze the non-transferred fertilized eggs (often called supernumeraries or additional embryos) for subsequent attempts. This procedure results in only one fresh embryo transfer, often undertaken in less than optimal conditions because of the ovarian status of hyper stimulation. The frozen embryos may serve in subsequent attempts, programmed close to the initial attempt in the case of implantation failure, or after parturition. In some cases, the frozen embryos are not reused because the couple has decided against transfer (they may feel they do not want any more children, or divorce or death may have intervened in the meantime). Currently, many frozen embryos are being conserved simply because the couple is undecided whether to proceed with another transfer or most often cannot face the decision to destroy them. In France, the couple legally has three alternatives: end the cryo-conservation of their embryos, allow early adoption by another couple facing a double sterility, or donate their embryos to research. (Paradoxically the law also forbids research on embryos conceived for that purpose.)

In Italy, a 2004 law (Legge N40) forbidding cryopreservation of the embryo forced resumption of work on oocyte freezing, with some encouraging results published by E. Porcu (Porcu et al., 1997). But even with modified slow-freezing in association with ICSI, results were not sufficient for the rest of Europe to follow suit. It was only after the publication of work by M. Kuwayama that IVF centres realized that oocyte freezing could be used in their practice. With rapid improvements in open system freezing, A. Cobo published results from a donor program showing that vitrified oocytes were equal in quality to fresh oocytes (Cobo et al., 2008, 2009). Because of their 2004 law, Italian teams realized that their situation was ideal to evaluate the efficiency of vitrification in an IVF program (Chamayou et al., 2006). Two major publications demonstrate the validity of the new procedure (Rienzi et al., 2010; Ubaldi et al., 2010). The embryo obtained with a vitrified/rewarmed oocyte has the same implantation rate as a fresh one demonstrated by L. Rienzi (Rienzi et al., 2010). Her report in Human Reproduction was the publication's most frequently downloaded work of the year 2011. A few months later F. Ubaldi from the same Roman team demonstrated that cumulative rates of pregnancy from the same cohort are equivalent to the cumulative rates from repeated attempts (Ubaldi et al., 2010). These publications underline the quality of the embryo produced from vitrification and its ability to implant. Oocyte vitrification will soon be widely adopted in IVF centres, as suggested in a recent meta-analysis review (Cobo & Diaz 2011). Each laboratory can decide to propose egg vitrification as an alternative to embryo freezing. In most centres employing micromanipulation, the technique itself is easily learned but its introduction in IVF programs requires some thought. Each centre will need to adopt its own strategy. In our centre we plan to conduct a study in which couples will be asked whether they prefer embryo or egg freezing, thus respecting their choice in the matter. It is expected some patients will still prefer to freeze their embryos, though once informed of the poorer implantation rates, they may decide to choose egg vitrification. (Currently in France, out of 100 births, 85 result from fresh transfer compared to 15 from thawing cycles.) We may of course modify our approach when comparative results for transfer of embryos produced from vitrified eggs are available on a large scale. Our study, to be conducted on the first couples for whom egg vitrification will be available in our centre (Boyer et al., 2009) is complementary to that of L. Rienzi (Rienzi et al., 2010). The benefit will be evaluated in terms of the probability of transfer for one selected oocyte. In a recent brief survey at our centre, half of the couples questioned said they would prefer oocyte freezing. We expect this proportion will increase when oocyte freezing becomes a real option.

In France, because the law prohibits research on human embryos produced for that purpose, research is conducted with embryos which for whatever reason have been rejected for human reproduction. This needs to be made clear to prospective parents (and to lawmakers as well).

2.1.1 The risk/reward balance of ovarian stimulation

Ovarian stimulation can proceed as usual; there will be no changes to the first step of IVF. We learn from the Italian experience that only 50% of the oocytes are of good quality, that is to say, appropriate for ICSI or vitrification. The first examination of the oocytes is crucial for a good result. An attempt at transfer will take place and the selected unused eggs will be vitrified for delayed microinjection. Egg banking schedules must take into account the number of couples who choose embryo freezing and also the number of embryos to be produced and transferred, as determined in our discussions with the couple. For transfers of embryos produced from vitrified oocytes, appointments will be based on the patient's menstrual cycle. In scheduling here we must be careful not to overload laboratory capacity.

An oocyte thawing cycle will be planned if the patient is not pregnant from the first transfer. Thawing of oocytes will be done 2 days after the LH surge or after triggering with hCG. All the cycles used for transfer will be free from ovarian stimulation risk. The natural cycle is preferred as it is the most favourable for embryo implantation.

The true challenge for centres offering an oocyte vitrification option will be scheduling the interventions. Clinicians must have a voice in the process. The laboratory calendar will have to take into account both fresh transfer and thawing cycles. If the natural cycle is most favourable for implantation, as has been reported, we will have to ensure that the laboratory can cope. The best day for the patient may not always be possible for the biologist!

2.1.2 Managing the oocyte cohort after pick-up

Centres must master the new procedure as developed by the leaders in the field, but for experienced biologists with skill in micromanipulation, the learning curve is not particularly steep. Within a very short time our centre was able to obtain oocytes or embryos of as good a quality as before vitrification and which, when transferred, resulted in ongoing pregnancies. (Fig 1, 2 and 3)

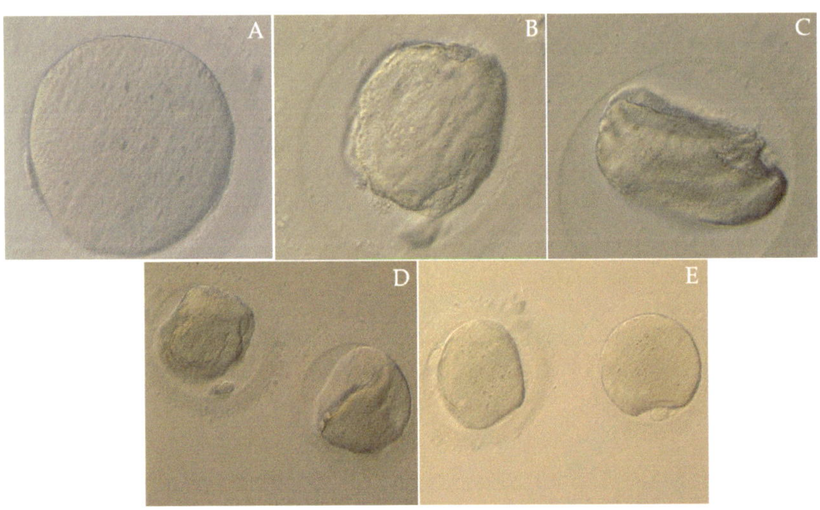

Fig. 1. Oocyte dehydration. In (A) the oocyte before dehydration begins. (B-D) the oocyte during dehydration: shrinkage. (E) the oocyte regaining original form with cryoprotectant filling.

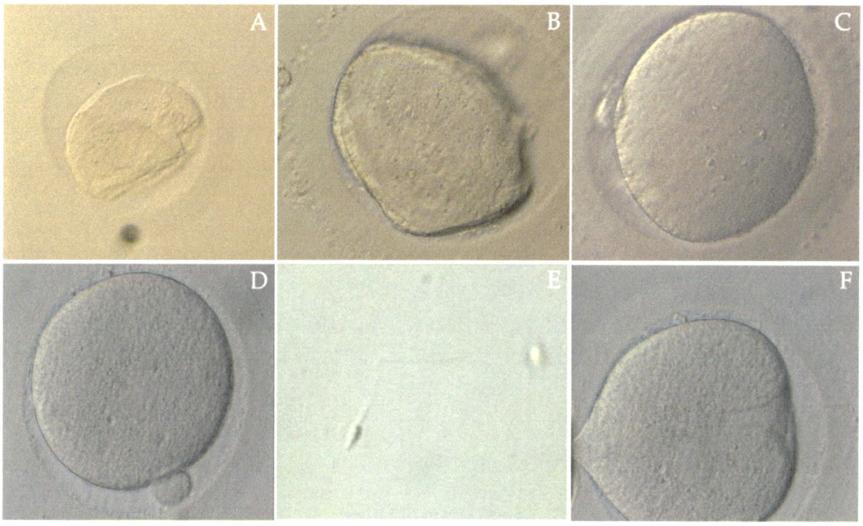

Fig. 2. Oocyte thawing and ICSI. (A-C) Oocyte shrinkage and re-gaining form during thawing. (D) Oocyte post-thawing. (E) Sperm selection for ICSI. (F) Oocyte post-ICSI.

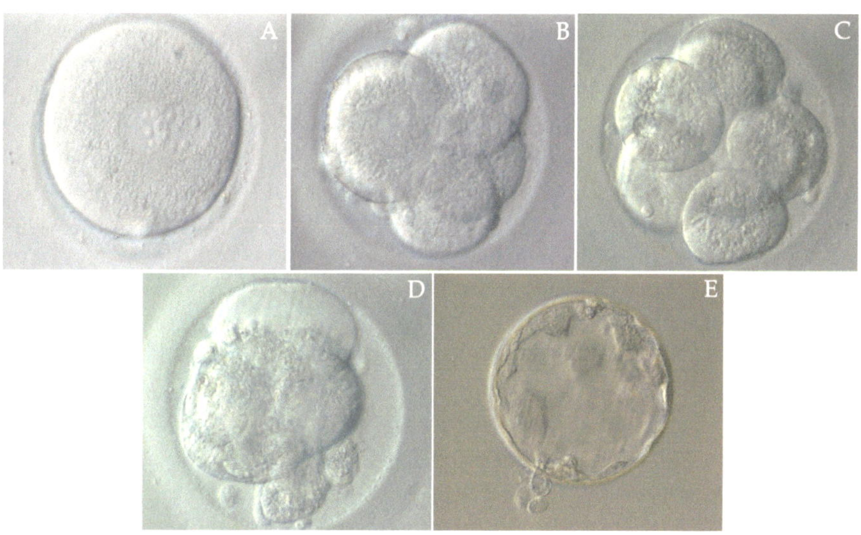

Fig. 3. Fresh oocyte development after vitrification, thawing and ICSI, identical to fresh oocytes development. (A) Zygote, day 1 in culture. (B) 4-cell embryo, day 2. (C) 8-cell embryo, day 3. (D) Morula, day 4. (E) Blastocyst, day 5.

The difficulty today remains deciding how many oocytes should be fertilized and how many vitrified. The daily practice of Italian teams and the results published in their annual report indicate that some 50% of the recovered oocytes are of good quality -- mature, in metaphase II, fertilizable and freezable. Based on their experience, it would be probably reasonable to propose 3 to 6 oocytes for fertilization, and vitrification of the rest. We can adjust these figures after some years of experience, as we did with ICSI. The number can be decided with each couple before starting the procedure. As a result we should be able to limit significantly the number of embryos produced as well as the number of frozen oocytes, without eliminating embryo freezing altogether.

After the denudation step, ICSI can be performed on part of the cohort as usual, followed by a fresh embryo transfer. The single embryo transfer is more frequent nowadays and the over-production of embryos is no longer necessary. The second portion of mature oocytes from the cohort can be vitrified for each patient. They will be used in a future attempt if the first embryo transfer has failed.

2.1.3 Overseeing the thawing of vitrified oocytes

As with single ovarian stimulation, most patients have more oocytes than they need for an embryo transfer. In more than half of all IVF cycles, there will be spare oocytes for at least one other fresh transfer, this time from the vitrified oocyte. For the second fresh transfer, the thawing of the selected oocytes must be scheduled early in the morning to allow for at least 2 hours in the incubator before fertilization. ICSI will be performed in all the surviving oocytes, with more than a 90 percent survival rate expected. Embryos are obtained and the transfer is organized as usual.

2.2 Impact on egg donation

Oocyte vitrification will have a major impact on egg donation by eliminating the complex coordination of donors and recipients. The need for synchronization between donor and recipient teams vanishes, simplifying all the steps necessary in preparing the donation. The creation of frozen egg banks will free us from the restraints which had previously limited our activity. Throughout the world, the mis-match between supply and demand has generated a lucrative business in which some of us have unfortunately become involved. Originally in almost all countries egg donation was developed for the altruistic purpose of providing healthy eggs to young women who for various reasons -- genetic, immunological, viral, and iatrogenic—were unable to produce them on their own. But in practice much of the demand has come from women who have turned to ART because of their age. Egg vitrification has opened the door to a new type of demand. A woman under 30 may now choose to preserve her fertility, even if she has no husband or plan for children at the time. Whether this possibility is a good thing is still matter of debate. However, we may legitimately ask if it is not better for a woman to preserve her own eggs at the age of 25 than to travel to a foreign country at the age of 45 to buy the eggs of young women there. Undoubtedly, we need to reflect on the implications of what has been termed "social egg freezing" (Lockwood, 2011). It is probably best to seek the answer from young women themselves rather than from bioethics committees whose members are often close to retirement. It is instructive in this regard to be in contact with teenage girls. We have often been surprised by their level of comfort with ART compared to older generations. The high cost of the new procedure poses problems of another order. With the advent of oocyte vitrification, the entire issue of egg donation will have to be re-evaluated, just as sperm donation had to be rethought when ICSI was first introduced.

2.2.1 How egg donation is currently organized

Young healthy women are asked to give their oocytes in return for some form of compensation, usually monetary. In most countries egg donors are first recruited. Synchronized cycles between recipient and donors are organized, eggs are shared with several recipients (depending on the number collected), and excess eggs are attributed to the recipient in case of implantation failure, resulting in super numerous embryos which are frozen even if the number is low (Boyer et al., 2010). One or more freezing/thawing cycles are usually included. With oocyte vitrification there is a risk we will see the explosive development of a market for oocytes especially in poor countries where young women have few opportunities for work and the payment is comparatively high (as with organ donation). We are facing a cross-border organization for egg donation where physicians in foreign countries compete to provide the most medically secure environment for the recipient. It is no secret that demand will come from patients over 40 in wealthier countries who have no other possibility of delivering successfully.

Over a period of ten years egg donation in Europe has increased more than three-fold, from 4500 cycles in 1998 to 15,000 in 2007, with half the donations coming from Spain. Even if the results -- a 60 percent pregnancy rate per cycle -- are good, the development of egg donations is worrisome because most patients are older women beyond the age of child-bearing. It is a flagrant example of the incursion of market practices in the medical profession. This problem is due to the nature of the demand but also to the growth of medical clinics run for financial profit. Biologists working in these clinics must reach goals set by financial directors. Health institutions today are guided more by financial considerations than medical. Today we see franchising of IVF units used as a tool to expand business. The unregulated European market has produced a situation which parallels the market worldwide, where certain practices migrate to countries with lower costs and/or looser regulation. Some centres propose an "all-in-one" stay that includes air tickets, hotel and on-site facilities. The world has seen a similar development in the fields of surrogacy, dentistry and cosmetic surgery.

2.2.2 How egg donation can be organized in a near future

The availability of unpaid oocytes is probably part of the solution. The possibility and quality of egg banking were assessed in a study by A. Cobo from IVI, presented at the ESHRE meeting in 2010 and published under the title, "A randomized, prospective, controlled-clinical trial to test the efficacy of oocyte banking in oocyte donation programs" (Cobo et al., 2010). This work, which demonstrates that ICSI using vitrified eggs produces the same results as with fresh recovered ones, marks a turning point in egg donation.

Oocyte vitrification makes in easier for each country to regulate its activity to fit the needs of its own population. Donations can be organized on a national scale, supervised by the health authorities of each country. Oocyte vitrification also will diversify the origin of donations. Oocytes from donors will be available but also from women who have undergone IVF treatment resulting in a successful pregnancy but who still have oocytes stored in the clinic where ICSI was performed and extra-numerary oocytes cryopreserved. Some of these women may agree to donate their "unused" oocytes to a national bank, and a national network can be organized. After some years of vitrified oocyte use, the number of eggs available for donation will tend to self-sufficiency.

2.3 Preventing loss of fertility

Female fertility is naturally limited to the years between puberty and menopause. The 15 best years are from the ages of 20 to 35. By the age of thirty, half of the oocytes available after birth have vanished (Gougeon et al., 1994, Faddy et al., 1995, Scheffer et al., 1999 Alviggi et al., 2009).

Oocyte freezing offers new possibilities for women who face loss of fertility either through familial risk or during medical treatment of serious pathologies (oncological diseases, etc.)

2.3.1 Identified familial or personal risk

When genetically-induced ovarian failure appears, it is often too late to preserve fertility because of the lack of oocytes, even if the woman is still young. However, the early prevention of fertility loss in patients with a known family history of premature infertility is possible. In some families, premature ovarian failure was identified in a woman's relatives who carried genetic mutations that interfere with the fertility timeline. In some cases a woman, although fertile at the age of 20, discovers she has lost her fertility ten years later, like her mother or aunt. In other cases, the discovery of the rearrangement of sex chromosomes may predict a shortened fertile life. It has been reported that carriers of Turner's syndrome can have their own oocytes in the early stages of the reproductive period (Haseltine et al., 1984).

By performing ovarian stimulation and collecting some oocytes while a woman still has antral follicles, it is possible to perform IVF later when she decides to use her eggs. Collecting them early in a woman's life can protect her from programmed premature menopause. With a few good oocytes, she maintains the possibility of bearing children later on.

2.3.2 Consequences of sterilizing treatments

Treatment for chronic or ontological diseases can affect a woman's fertility, partially or definitively. In almost all such cases, survival and cure rates are high and the woman is young enough to conceive after recovery. In the past ten years, the medical focus for such patients has been the cryopreservation of cortical fragments of the ovaries, and the programming of a graft for a hormonal ovarian cycle recovery. In rare cases an attempted pregnancy has been suggested to restore fertility. Some births have been reported but remain low due to the difficulties of the surgical procedure (Roux et al., 2010). By vitrifying oocytes in some women who are able to undergo ovarian stimulation before treatment, preservation of fertility will be more efficient (Porcu et al., 2008, Noyes et al., 2011). The new method provides a better alternative for women facing loss of sterility through treatment of certain diseases.

2.3.3 Embryo freezing has new rival for preserving female fertility

However, the most interesting prospect offered by oocyte vitrification is societal -- it is now possible to avoid cryopreservation of the embryo. Many prominent bodies have argued that cryopreservation of the embryo is safe and efficient, thus legitimizing its use for the preservation of woman's fertility. This has been the position of the American Society for Reproductive Medicine (Practice Committee of ASRM 2008), the French College of Gynaecology and Obstetrics (Bringer et al., 2010) and probably that of many other countries. We regard this as a true mistake. Take the case of the Evans couple which was brought before the European Court of Human Rights (European Court of Human Rights 2006). In 2000 the Evans were faced with a difficult situation. Mrs Evans was diagnosed with an ovarian tumour. They were advised by medical staff to proceed with IFV as a couple, and as a result six embryos were obtained and cryopreserved. The couple later divorced and Mrs Evans was denied use of the embryos. Mr Evans would not consent to an embryo transfer. She took her case to the European Court of Human Rights which ruled in her former husband's favour. The position of the European Court was that his right to withdraw consent was stronger than her right to use the embryos without his consent. For Mrs Evans it was a double condemnation -- her ability to have her own children was taken away, first through illness and again by the courts. With oocyte vitrification such an outcome could have been avoided, because she would have been sole owner of her eggs.

It should also be noted that the current debate over the future of unused embryos could become irrelevant. Should they be destroyed? Given to another couple? Is it legitimate to refuse embryo transfer post-mortem? Or to accept post-mortem transfer but within certain time limits? And if so, how long after death? And how many transfers should be allowed? As long as the preservation of embryos is the preferred method, these issues will continue to plague societies.

A few years ago in the French city of Toulouse a woman was refused an embryo transfer because her husband (the "father") was no longer alive. The court ruled that her embryos be proposed for "very early adoption" because of a 2004 law in France prohibiting destruction of human embryos.

Today, we are no longer being forced to choose between the right to motherhood and the right not to become father. Women are now able to preserve their gametes. Oocyte vitrification will resolve a number of ethical issues surrounding the use of the human embryo, without creating new dilemmas. We must be prepared at some point to admit our error in promoting embryo freezing as a means of preserving fertility and recognize that this is not a minor issue.

As underlined by Cobo, the American Society for Reproductive Medicine concludes, "Oocyte cryopreservation presently should be considered an experimental technique only to be performed under investigational protocol under the auspices of an Institutional Review Board." The French College of Gynaecologists et Obstetricians reaches a similar conclusion. All such professional organizations have a duty to rectify their position, once proof of error has been reasonably established.

3. Conclusion

The time has come to reorganize our daily practice, integrating oocyte vitrification into our routines. The efficiency of the combined techniques of ICSI and oocyte vitrification has transformed our environment, necessitating the creation of cryobiology units in all our labs where that has not already been done. We may rejoice in this recognition of our speciality in the field of medicine. We must continue to form a new generation of specialists, in a professional world very different from what we once knew. In over 30 years of practice we have been witness every ten years to major changes in the field. We must share our experience with the new generation, while hoping fervently they will have the freedom to follow. In today's often oppressive regulatory environment, practitioners are caught up in concerns over quality control, their CE mark and ISO15189 accreditation. We will lose our souls this way. Regulatory pressures have led not only to modifications of all our procedures, they have transformed the structural functioning of our units. As biologists we must reassert our control in the lab. We cannot delegate the most critical aspects of our procedures to technicians who lack the understanding to take medical decisions.

The advent of oocyte vitrification, like the introduction of ICSI before, poses a real challenge. This challenge will be met with success by all those who have chosen to dedicate their lives to reproductive biology. We are on the threshold of a cryobiological revolution. We can preserve oocytes today. In the future we will be able to preserve entire organs. We are fortunate to be working in this amazing field; may we remain passionate about our true mission -- to help patients. The introduction of oocyte vitrification represents a major step in the field of reproductive biology. It will transform our procedures, curtail the cryopreservation of embryos and resolve many issues surrounding the status of the human embryo. The advances are medical but they will have broad political, social and legal impact as well.

4. References

Al-Hasani, S.; Ozmen, B.; Koutlaki, N. ; Schoepper, B.; Diedrich, K. & Schultze-Mosgau, A (2007) Three years of routine vitrification of human zygotes: is it still fair to advocate slow-rate freezing? *Reprod BioMed Online* 14: 288-93

Alviggi, C.; Humaidan, P.; Howles,; C.; Treway, D. & Hillier, S. Biological versus chronological ovarian age: implications for assisted reproductionreproductive technology. (2009) Reprod. Biol. Endoc. 7: 1-13

Balaban, B.; Urman, B.; Ata, B.; Isiklar, A.; Larman, M.; Hamilton, R. & Gardner, D. (2008) A randomized controlled study of human Day 3 embryo cryopreservation by slow freezing or vitrification: vitrification is associated with higher survival, metabolism and blastocyst formation *Hum. Reprod.* 23 (9): pp1976-1982

Bielanski A, & Vajta G. (2009) Risk of contamination of germplasm during cryopreservation and cryobanking in IVF units. *Hum Reprod.* 24 (10) pp. 2457-67.

Boyer, P.; Gervoise-Boyer, M.; Tourame, P.; Poirot, C. & Le Coz, P. (2009) Information sur une nouvelle technique : la vitrification des ovocytes. *Bull. Acad. Natl. Méd.* 193: 1113-25

Boyer, P.; Tourame, P. & Le Coz, P. Nouvelles techniques d'Assistance médicale à la procréation: la France aux abonnés absents. Lettre ouverte sur la vitrification ovocytaire (2010) *Gynecol. Obstet. Fertil.* 2010, 38, (10), pp. 561-562

Boyer, P.; Gervoise-Boyer, M.; Tourame, P.; Le Coz, P. & Poirot; C. Réponse. à l'article de F. Merlet et B. Senemaud : « prise en charge du don d'ovocytes : règlementation du don, la face cachée du tourisme procréatif » (2010) *Gynecol. Obstet. Fertil;* 38: pp 36–44.

Bringer-Deutsch, S.; Belaisch-Allart, J. & Delvigne, A. (2010) Préservation de la fertilité en cas de traitement stérilisant. *J. Gyn. Obst. Biol; Repod,* 39 S53-66

Chamayou, S.; Alecci, C. ; Ragolia, C.; Storaci, G.; Maglia, E.; Russo, E.; & Guglielmino, A. (2006) Comparison of in-vitro outcomes from cryopreserved oocytes and sibling fresh oocytes. *Reprod Biomed Online* 12: 779–96

Chen, C. Pregnancy after human oocyte cryopreservation. (1986) *Lancet i* : 884-6.

Chian, R.; Huang, J.; Tan, S.; Lucena, E.; Saa, A.; Rojas, A.; Castellón, L.; Amador, M. & Sarmiento, J. (2008) Obstetric and perinatal outcome in 200 infants conceived from vitrified oocytes. *Reprod. Biomed. Online* 16: 608-10

Cobo, A.; Kuwayama, M.; Perez, S.; Ruiz, A.; Pellicer, A. & Remohí, J. (2008) Comparison of concomitant outcome achieved with fresh and cryopreserved donor oocytes vitrified by the Cryotop method. *Fertil. Steril.* 89:1657-64

Cobo, A.; Vajta, G. & Remohí, J. (2009) Vitrification of human mature oocytes in clinical practice. *Reprod Biomed Online* 19: Suppl 4

Cobo, A.; Meseguer, M.; Remohı, J. & Pellicer, A. (2010) Use of cryo-banked oocytes in an ovum donation programme: a prospective, randomized, controlled, clinical trial *Hum. Reprod.* 25 (9) pp. 2239–2246

Cobo, A. & Diaz, C. Clinical application of oocyte vitrification: a systematic review and meta-analysis of randomizes controlled trials. (2011) *Fertil. Steril.* 96: 277-85

Cutting, R.; Barlow, S. & Anderson, R. (2009) Human oocyte cryopreservation: evidence for practice. Association of Clinical Embryologists and British Fertility Society. *Hum Fertil* 12: 125-36

Dessolle, L.; Biau, D.; Larouzière, V.; Ravel, C.; Antoine, J.; Daraï, E. & Mandelbaum, J. (2009) Learning curve of vitrification assessed by cumulative summation test for learning curve (LC-CUSUM) *Fertil. Steril.* (92) pp: 943-945

European Court of Human Rights, Fourth Section, Case of Evans v. The United Kingdom, Application no. 63339/05, 7 mars 2006, § 65

Faddy,M. & Gosden, R. (1995) A mathematical model of follicular dynamics in the human ovary. *Hum. Reprod.* 10 pp 770-5

Fadini, R.; Brambillasca, F.; Renzini, M.; Merola, M.; Comi, R. & De Ponti Dal Canto E. (2009) Human oocyte cryopreservation: comparison between slow and ultra-rapid methods. *Reprod BioMed Online* 19: pp171-180

Gougeon, A.; Echocard, R. & Thalabard, J. (1994) Age-related changes of the population of human ovarian follicles: increase in the disappearance rate of non-growing and early-growing follicles in aging women. *Biol. Reprod.* 50 pp 653-63

Gook, D. & Edgar D. Human oocyte cryopreservation. (2007) *Hum Reprod Update,* 13: pp 591-605.

Kuleshova, L.; Gianaroli, L.; Magli, C.; Ferraretti, A. & Trounson, A. (1999) Birth following vitrification of a small number of human oocytes: case report *Hum. Reprod.* (1999) 14 (12): 3077-3079.

Kuwayama, M. Highly efficient vitrification for cryopreservationof human oocytes and embryos: the Cryotop method. (2007) *Theriogenology* 67: pp 73–80.

Legge contenente norme in materia di Procreazione Medicalemente Assistita. (2008) Legge 19 febbraio 2004, N 40, Articulo 15

Lockwood, G. (2011) Social egg freezing: the prospect of reproductive "immortality" or dangerous delusion, *Reprod. Biomed Online* 23: pp 334-40

Mukaida, T.; Takahashi, K.; Goto, T. & Oka, C. (2009) Perinatal outcome of vitrified human blastocyst in 9 years experience (3 601 cycles) including the incidence rate of monozygote twinning. *Hum. Reprod.* 24: i28

Nagy, Z.; Chang, C.; Shapiro, D.; Bernal, D.; Elsner, C.; Mitchell-Leef, D.; Toledo, A. & Kort,., (2009). Clinical evaluation of the efficiency of an oocyte donation program using egg cryo-banking. *Fertil. Steril.* 92, 520–526.

Noyes, N.; Porcu, E. & Borini, A. (2009) Over 900 oocyte cryopreservation babies born with no apparent increase in congenital anomalies. *Reprod. Biomed Online* 18: pp 769-76

Noyes, N.; Knopman, J.; Melzer, K.; Fino, E.; Fiedman, & Westphal, L. Oocyte cryopreservation as a fertility preservation measure for cancer patients. (2011) *Reprod Biomed Online* 23: pp 3232-33

Paffoni, A.; Guarneri, C.; Ferrari,,S.; Restelli, L.; Nicolosi, A.; Scarduelli, C. & Ragni, G. Effects of two vitrification protocols on the developmental potential of human mature oocytes (2011) *Reprod. Biomed. Online* 22: pp 292- 298

Palermo, G.; Joris, H.; Devroey, P. & Van Steirteghem, A. (1992) Pregnancies after intracytoplasmic injection of single spermatozoon into an oocyte *Lancet* (340) 8810 pp 17-18

Parmegiani, L.; Accorsi, A.; Cognigni, G.; Bernardi, S.; Troilo, E. & Filicori, M. (2010) Sterilization of liquid nitrogen with ultravioletirradiation for safe vitrification of human oocytes or embryos *Fertil. Steril.* 94: pp.1525–8.

Porcu, E.; Fabbri, R.; Seracchioli, R.; Ciotti, P.; Magrini, O. & Flamigni, C. (1997) Birth of a healthy female after intracytoplasmic sperm injection of cryopreserved human oocytes *Fertil. Steril.* 68: pp 724-726

Porcu, E.; Bazzocchi. A.; Notarangelo. L.; Paradisi, R.; Landolfo, C. & Venturoli, S. (2008) Human oocyte cryopresvervation in infertility and oncololy *Review. Curr Opin Endocrinol Diabetes Obes* 15: 529-35

Practice Committee of American Society for Reproductive Medicine; Practice Committee of Society for Assisted Reproductive Technology. Ovarian tissue and oocyte cryopreservation. *Fertil. Steril.* 2008;90: S241-6.

Relazione del Ministro della Salute al Parlamento sullo stato di Attuazione della legge contenente norme in materia di procreazione medicalmente assistita (legge 19 febbraio 2004, n. 40, articolo 15) - anno 2009 Anno di pubblicazione: 2011

Rienzy, L.; Romano, S.; Albricci, L.; Maggiulli, R.; Capalbo, A.; Baroni, E.; Colamaria, S.; Sapienza, F. & Ubaldi, F. (2010) Embryo development of fresh *versus* vitrified metaphase II oocytes after ICSI: a prospective randomized sibling-oocytestudy. *Hum. Reprod.* 25: 66-73

Roux, C.; Amiot, C.; Agnani, G. Aubart, Y. ; Rohrlich, P. &Pivert, P. (2010) Live birth after ovarian tissue autograft in a patient with sickle cell disease treated by allogeneic bone marrow transplantation *Fertil. Steril.* 93 pp 2413

Scheffer, G.; Broelmans, J.; Dorland, M.; Habbema, J.; Looman, C. & de Velde E. (1999) Antral follicule counts by transvaginal ultrasonography are related to age in women with proven natural fertility. *Fertil. Steril.* 72: pp 845-51

Smith, G.; Serafin, P.; Fioravanti, J.;. Yaid, I.; Coslovsky, M.; Hassum, P.; Alegretti, R.; & Motta, E. (2010) Prospective randomized comparison of human oocytes cryopreservation with slow-rate freezing or vitrification *Fertil. Steril.* (94): pp2088-2095

Steptoe, P.; & Edwards, R. (1978). Birth after the reimplantation of a human embryo. *Lancet* ii (8085), 366.

Takahashi, K.; Mukaida, T.; Goto, T. & Oka, C. (2005) Perinatal outcome of blastocyst transfer with vitrification using cryoloop: a 4-year follow-up study. *Fertil Steril* 84: 88-92

Tao, T.; Zhang, W.; & Del Valle, A. (2009) Review. Human oocyte cryopreservation. *Curr Opin Obstet Gynecol.* 21: 247-52

Trokoudes, M. ; Pavlides, K. & Zhang, X. (2011) Comparison outcome of fresh and vitrified donor oocytes in an egg-sharing donation program *Fertil. Steril.*95, (6) 6 , pp1996-2000,

Trounson, A.;. & Mohr, L. Human pregnancy following cryopreservation,thawing and transfer of an eight-cell embryo.(1983). *Nature* 305, 707-709.

Ubaldi, F.; Anniballo, R.; Romano, S.; Baroni, E.; Albricci, L.; Colamaria, S.; Capalbol, A.; Vajta, G. & Rienzy, L. (2010) Cumulative ongoing pregnancy rate achieved with oocyte vitrification and cleavage stage transfer without embryo selection in a standard infertility program. *Hum. Reprod.* 25 (5), 1199-1205.

Vanderzwalmen, P.; Ebner, T. & Zech, N. (2007) One decade of experience with vitrification of human embryos in straws, hemi-straws and high security vitrification straws. In: *Vitrification in Assisted Reproduction, a user's Manual and Trouble - Shooting Guide.* INFORMA Healthcare, pp. 195-217, Edit, London

Vajta, G. & Nagy, Z. (2009) Are programmable freezers still needed in the embryo laboratory? Review on vitrification. *Reprod Biomed Online* 19: Suppl 4

Wennerholm, U.; Söderström-Anttila, V.; Bergh, C.; Aittomäki, K.; Nygren, K.; Selbing, A. & Loft, A. (2009) Children born after cryopreservation of embryos or oocytes: a systematic review of outcome data. *Hum Reprod.* 24: 2158-72

8

Preimplantation Genetic Testing: Current Status and Future Prospects

Eduardo C. Lau[1], Marleen M. Janson[1], Carl B. Ball[1,2], Mark R. Roesler[3], Peter VanTuinen[1], David P. Bick[1,4] and Estil Y. Strawn[1,3]

[1] *Medical College of Wisconsin,*
[2]*Alverno College,*
[3]*Froedtert Hospital,*
[4]*Children's Hospital of Wisconsin*
USA

1. Introduction

While *in vitro* fertilization (IVF) is most often employed as a remedy for infertility, a discussion of the field would not be complete if it did not address the application of IVF to avoid genetic disorders. IVF makes it possible to assess the genetic status of the embryo before establishing a pregnancy when couples are at risk for an affected child. Physicians in the field will benefit from being informed about the diverse set of molecular and cytogenetic technologies employed in preimplantation genetic diagnosis (PGD) and screening (PGS), and from understanding their relative power and limitations as tools for genetic counseling.

PGD and pre-implantation genetic screening (PGS) refer to two distinct types of clinical procedure that help a couple to have a healthy child: PGD determines the embryo's genotype, while PGS assesses an embryo's karyotype and has been used in screening chromosomal aneuploidy.

PGD and PGS require the use of the IVF technique. These technologies, initiated in the late 1980s as an alternative to prenatal diagnosis (PND), allows a couple at risk of a genetic disorder to give birth to an unaffected child by avoiding selective termination of an affected pregnancy. Genetic disorders could be due to either a single gene disorder, or an abnormal number or structure of chromosomes. The current agreed upon indications (Cooper & Jungheim, 2010) for PGD and PGS include:

1. Screening for embryo chromosomal aneuploidy in cases of advanced maternal age or known parental translocation
2. Family history indicating risk for known autosomal Mendelian genetic disorders
3. Sex selection with family history indicating risk for X-linked disorders
4. Sex selection for family balancing, e.g. parental preference for a male or female
5. Human leukocyte antigen (HLA) matching to achieve a child to provide hematopoietic progenitor cells from cord blood to an existing sibling who requires bone marrow transplantation

The medical need for these services is significant. The U.S. Centers for Disease Control and Prevention estimates that more than 6,000 single-gene disorders affect approximately 1 in 300 live-births (Benson and Haith, 2009), while cytogenetic abnormalities appear at about twice this rate in live births and cause approximately ¼ of miscarriages and stillbirths (Thiesen & Shaffer, 2010). PGD makes it possible to assess the genetic status of at-risk embryos prior to implantation and initiation of a potentially affected pregnancy. There still remains considerable controversy regarding the need for and the ability of PGD to increase implantation rates for IVF.

1.1 The milestones of PGD and PGS development

PGD began in the late 1980's with the pioneering work by Handyside and colleagues in selecting embryo gender by polymerase chain reaction (PCR) amplification (Handyside et al., 1990), and diagnosis for a recessive autosomal disorder (Handyside et al., 1992).

PGS was subsequently developed by Munne's team for gender determination (Munne et al., 1993), and by Handyside's team for aneuploidy screening (Schrurs et al., 1993) using fluorescent in-situ hybridization (FISH). Other PGD milestones include its application for chromosomal translocations (Munne et al., 1998), and for HLA matching that led to the first HLA matched baby unaffected with Fanconi anemia (Verlinsky et al., 2001; Grewal et al., 2004).

Between the birth of the first PGD baby in 1989 and the year 2000, about 500 babies were born worldwide using PGD. Since then, the PGD has been on a steep rise: about 1000 PGD babies were born worldwide between 2000 and 2002, and 1500 more PGD babies were born between 2002 and 2004 (Verlinsky et al., 2004; ESHRE PGD Consortium, 2002; Harper et al., 2010). In the past 21 years, while thousands of babies have been born following PGD, there are no confirmed reports of increased fetal abnormalities following PGD.

1.2 Assisted reproductive technologies that support preimplanation genetic testing

Preimplementation genetic testing is supported by advances in assisted reproductive technology (ART). Methodologies of particular importance include intracytoplasmic sperm injection (ICSI), laser-assisted biopsies of embryos at the cleavage and blastocyst stages, sperm sorting, and cryopreservation of biopsied embryos.

1.2.1 Intracytoplasmic sperm injection

In conventional IVF each egg is combined with several thousand motile sperms on the day of egg retrieval to fertilize the egg. As a result, numerous sperms are present around the fertilized egg. At the next step, embryo biopsy, these excess sperms can contaminate the biopsy and contamination of the embryonic sample with sperm DNA can lead to incorrect PGD results. To guard against this risk a single sperm can be injected into each egg. This procedure is known as intracytoplasmic sperm injection (ICSI; Palermo et al., 1992; Harton et al., 2011a).

Through ICSI eggs are fertilized and embryos are formed. On day 3 of fertilization, a single blastomere is removed from each cleavage-stage embryo having 6-8 cells for PGD. When embryos develop into blastocysts on day 5 of fertilization, embryos selected by PGD are transferred to the mother. Alternatively, a few cells can be removed from the trophectoderm of a blastocyst for PGD on day 5, but the embryo will need to be transferred on day 6. Otherwise, the blastocysts need to be stored frozen and transferred at the next fertilization cycle.

1.2.2 Laser-assisted biopsy of embryos

PGD is accomplished by evaluating genetic material in polar bodies from unfertilized and fertilized oocytes (not performed here), blastomeres from cleavage-stage embryos, or trophectoderm cells from blastocysts. Depending on the developmental stage (oocyte, embryo or blastocyst), the zona pellucida can be breeched by one of three methods: mechanical zona drilling, acidified Tyrodes solution or laser.

At present, the cleavage stage is most widely used for embryo biopsy, and drilling a hole in the zona pellucida with a laser beam is the predominant method (Harton et al., 2011b). On day 3 of fertilization when normally developing embroys reach the 8-cell stage, one or two blastomeres are aspirated through the opening of a cleavage-stage embryo for PGD using a glass capillary pipette. This is also known as blastomere biopsy.

Biopsy of embryos at the blastocyst stage (on day 5 of fertilization) is more technically demanding (Fig. 1). An advantage of blastocyst biopsy is that this procedure is noninvasive

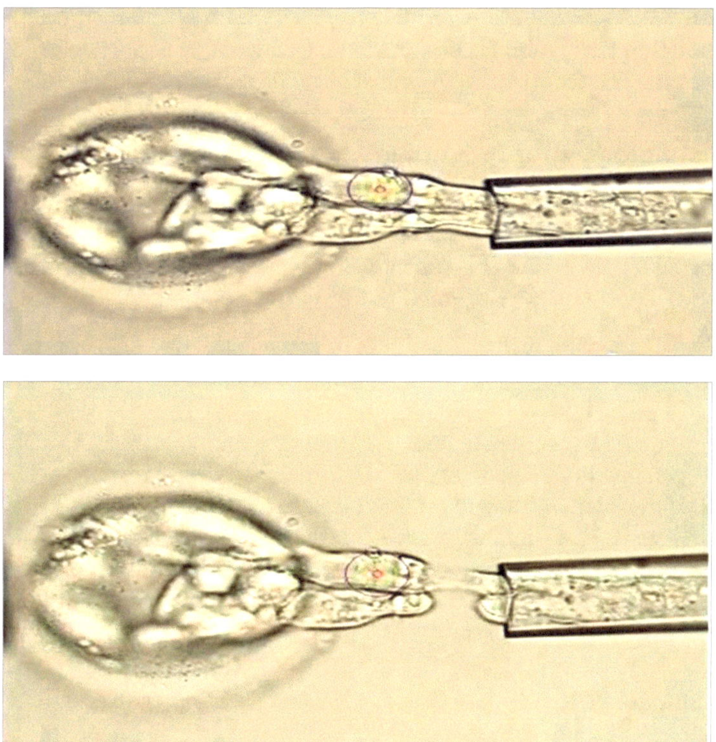

Fig. 1. Laser-assisted blastocyst biopsy. Shown in the *top* and *bottom* panels *before* and *after* the removal of a few trophectoderm cells from an embryo at the blastocyst stage for PGD, respectively. On day 5 post-fertilization, a few cells excised from the trophectoderm by laser beam are aspirated using a glass capillary pipette under stereo microscope.

to the inner cell mass of the embryo because cells are removed only from the trophectoderm that will become the placenta. A further advantage is that the removal of multiple cells for PGD will significantly lower the allele drop-out (ADO) rate and increase the accuracy of testing. A drawback of blasocyst testing is that it allows less time for PGD, and thus the embryo may need to be frozen for transfer in the next fertilization cycle if test results are not obtained within a day.

1.2.3 Sperm sorting

After binding non-intercalating fluorescent dye to their DNA, X- and Y-bearing sperms are separated by flow-activated cell sorting based on the difference in total DNA content. The purity is greater than 70% for Y-bearing sperms, but greater than 90% for X-bearing sperms. Sperm sorting can be used for preconception sex selection used in family balancing, or used in combination with IVF-PGD to prevent the transmission of X-linked recessive diseases.

1.2.4 Cryopreservation of biopsied embryos at the blastocyst stage

Using the standard freeze-thaw method, the survival rate is low when cleavage-stage embryos (on day 3 of fertilization) are biopsied and cryopreserved. The survival rate can, however, be improved by vitrification after incubating the cleavage-stage embryos for 6-8 h following biopsy (Zheng et al., 2005), or by cryopreservation in CJ3 medium (Stachecki et al., 2005). Recently higher survival rates of biopsied cleavage-stage embryos have been obtained by vitrification at the blastocyst stage (Magli et al., 2006; Zhang et al., 2009).

2. Current technologies for preimplantation genetic testing

At the Medical College of Wisconsin and Froedtert Hospital (Milwaukee, Wisconsin, U.S.A.) we provide PGD and PDS services for medically indicated conditions (Bick & Lau, 2006; Swanson et al, 2007). PGS for chromosomal aneuploidies (monosomy or trisomy) and chromosomal translocations is performed by FISH (Swanson et al., 2007). We also provide PGD for HLA matching (Bick et al., 2008), diagnosis of specific single-gene disorders (Swanson et al., 2007; Lau et al., 2010), and gender selection in cases of X-linked diseases (E.C. Lau, K. Wang & M.M. Janson, unpublished).

For a family with a child who needs bone marrow transplantation, PGD for HLA matching (tissue typing) can facilitate birth of an HLA-matched donor infant (Bick et al., 2008; Verlinsky et al., 2001). Hematopoietic progenitor cells are then transplanted from cord blood or bone marrow of the PGD infant to save the life of the affected sibling. In addition, we have developed PGD assays for a few common and/or severe childhood genetic diseases, such as spinal muscular atrophy, sickle cell anemia, autosomal recessive polycystic kidney disease (ARPKD), and cystic fibrosis.

2.1 PGD by multiplex PCR

Single-cell multiplex PCR has been used in the PGD assays for HLA matching, spinal muscular atrophy (SMA) and sickle cell anemia. In PGD for these disorders we perform multiplex PCR of single blastomeres followed by haplotyping analysis of embryos with several linked short tandem repeat (STR) markers (Bick et al., 2008). Multiple markers are used due to the high incidence of allele-drop-out for single-cell PCR.

In PGD for SMA, we perform multiplex nested PCR of single blastomeres followed by restriction cleavage analysis (Swanson et al., 2007). This technique detects the restriction fragment length polymorphisms (RFLPs) of the *SMN1* and *SMN2* genes at exons 7 and 8. We use Hinf I for cleaving exon 7 (Daniels et al., 2001), and Dde I for cleaving exon 8 of the *SMN* genes (Malcov et al., 2004). We use both fast PCR reaction mixture and rapid restriction enzymes to shorten the turn-around-time of PGD for SMA (E.C. Lau, unpublished). SMA, an autosomal recessive motor neuron disorder, is the most common fatal genetic disorder in childhood. It affects 1 in 6,000 to 1 in 10,000 live births, and has carrier frequency of 1 in 40 to 1 in 60 in the population. Deletion of both copies of *SMN1* gene accounts for 95% of SMA cases. *SMN2* gene is highly homologous to *SMN1*, but cannot substitute for *SMN1* gene functions (Prior & Russman, 2011).

In PGD for sickle cell anemia, we perform multiplex PCR of single blastomeres followed by detection of β-globin (*HBB*) gene mutations by mini-sequencing, which is also known as single-base primer extension (Kobayashi et al., 1995; Heinrich et al., 2009). Sickle cell anemia is an autosomal recessive disorder caused by single-base mutation in codon 6 of *HBB* gene, that substitutes a thymine for adenine. A conformational change in the hemoglobin S (Hb S) molecule reduces its ability to carry oxygen. Other types of sickle cell diseases result from co-inheritance of HbS with abnormal globin β-chain variants, such as sickle hemoglobin C disease (Hb SC), and sickle β-thalassemia. In PGD for sickle cell diseases, linkage analysis of *HBB* haplotypes is performed with linked STRs located within the *HBB* gene and its flanking regions (E.C. Lau, A.F. Licht & M.M. Janson, unpublished).

The major drawback of PGD by multiplex PCR is the interaction of PCR primers, which results in a long and tedious optimization process to work out a robust mixture for each patient family (see Section 3.1).

2.2 PGD by whole-genome amplification

A major challenge of PGD is to amplify DNA from single blastomeres and perform genotyping analysis within the time constraints of the IVF cycle. In order to meet the turn-around-time of 30 hours or less for PGD from receiving the biopsied cells to clinical report, we have developed a fast and reliable protocol for whole-genome amplification (WGA) from single cells using multiple displacement amplification (MDA; Lau et al., 2010). Amplification is necessary since a single cell does not contain enough DNA to fulfill these assays.

2.2.1 Techniques for single-cell whole-genome amplification

The earliest method for whole-genome amplification (WGA) from single cells was PCR-based primer-extension preamplification (PEP) of single sperms (Zhang et al. 1992), that was adapted for the amplification of single blastomeres in PGD (Sermon et al., 1996). Like other PCR-based methods for WGA, the drawbacks of PEP method were incomplete genome coverage, and amplification bias (10^3 to 10^6 folds) between genomic loci in amplified products.

More recent technologies for WGA from single cells are multiple displacement amplification (MDA; Handyside et al., 2004; Lau et al., 2010; Dean et al., 2002) and PicoPlex® library methods. MDA is a non-PCR and isothermal method for DNA amplification. Handyside and colleagues used a commercial MDA kit to amplify single blastomeres for PGD (Handyside et al., 2004; Hellani et al., 2004), but the reaction time was 16 hours, and the ADO rates for genotyping MDA products were as high as 34%. While commercial kits for MDA are optimized for greater than 10 ng input genomic DNA, the use of MDA for WGA of single cells is not a standard application supported by the kit manufacturers (Coskun & Alsmadi, 2007). We modified the reaction of a commercial rapid-MDA kit for single cells, and obtained genotyping results of less than 10% ADO after 4-h MDA reaction (Lau et al., 2010).

An alternative method for WGA from single cells is the PicoPlex® kit, which is adapted from the OmniPlex® technique for genomic DNA (Langmore 2002). The PicoPlex® library kit for WGA is a PCR-based technique that requires the fragmentation of large genomic DNA prior to the construction of a PCR-amplifiable library. Both MDA and PicoPlex® methods for single-cell WGA have been used in array-based preimplantation testing (Hellani et al., 2008; Johnson et al., 2010; see Section 3.1).

2.2.2 Linkage approach for embryo analysis

Besides direct mutation detection, we use a linkage approach for embryo and familial analysis in PGD. For PGD of single-gene disorders, genotyping analysis is performed for embryos using STR markers linked with the disease genes, followed by haplotyping analysis.

"Preimplantation genetic haplotyping" (PGH) is a test procedure for which the first round is whole genome amplification (WGA) of single blastomeres, and the second round is genotyping using whole-genome amplified products as template. A comparison of sizes and genotypes of STRs among family members allows inferences of the haplotypes for parents and an affected child. If the STR loci are closely linked to and flank the disease locus, unaffected embryos can be identified by comparing their haplotypes to those of the parents and affected sibling. The advantage of using single-cell WGA in the first round of PGD is that a single common protocol is used to make many copies of the entire genome for subsequent analysis.

We have successfully applied PGH to PGD for single-gene recessive disorders, such as autosomal recessive polycystic kidney disease (ARPKD; Lau et al. 2010) and cystic fibrosis (E.C. Lau, M.M. Janson & T. Boyle, unpublished). ARPKD is caused by mutations in the *PKHD1* gene, which is located at chromosome 6p12.2 and codes for fibrocystin protein. Although 2-5% of all cases of polycystic kidney diseases (PKD) are ARPKD, more than 75% of all PKD cases that present clinically in the first month of life are ARPKD, with a mortality rate of about 25% in the first month of life (Sweeney & Avner, 2006; Dell & Avner, 2008). ARPKD affects approximately 1 in 20,000 live-births, with a carrier frequency of 1 in 70 individuals. The first PGD case for a family at risk for autosomal recessive polycystic kidney disease (ARPKD) was successful using PGH (Lau et al., 2010). A PGD child, whose sibling died at birth from the disease and whose parents were both carriers of the gene, was born healthy with normal kidneys.

We have also applied the PGH approach to PGD for cystic fibrosis (CF). CF is the most common lethal autosomal recessive disorder among Caucasians of northern European ancestry, and is a common genetic cause of infant mortality. The carrier frequency among Caucasians in the United States is approximately 1 in 25, but is lower in other racial groups. Over 1,000 different mutations in the *CFTR* gene for CF have been described, but fewer than 25 occur with appreciable frequency (Amos et al. 2006).

PGD for single-gene disorders by PGH is a general approach based on linkage analysis. It does not require prior knowledge of the exact nucleotide sites of the mutations within a gene. PGH saves the time required to develop custom PGH assays for individual alleles, and thus is particularly useful for PGD of single-gene disorders involving many rare or private mutations. However, the haplotyping approach for PGD also has limitations. The method would be unable to determine the parental haplotypes when the affected child is deceased and a DNA specimen is unavailable. In addition, PGH will not infer the correct parental haplotypes if the affected inherited a chromosome that had undergone recombination at the disease locus (Altarescu et al., 2008).

2.3 PGD for gender selection

The application of PGD for gender selection offers an alternative to single-gene assays for individual X-linked diseases. Instead of developing custom PGD assays for individual X-linked diseases, it is more practical to provide a single PGD assay of gender identification for families at risk of X-linked diseases. To prevent the transmission of X-linked Mendelian recessive diseases, PGD is used to select female embryos offspring. Because two copies of the mutant X allele are required for the diseases to occur in females, daughters of unaffected fathers will at worst be carriers for the trait. By contast, in males only one copy of the mutant X allele is required for the disease to occur and so the male child of a carrier mother has a 50% risk of having the disease.

2.3.1 Applications of PGD for gender selection

The main medical use of PGD for gender selection is to prevent the transmission of X-linked Mendelian recessive disorders by giving birth to female offspring. Many X-linked Mendelian recessive disorders, such as Duchenne muscular dystrophy (DMD), and hemophilia A and B, are rarely seen in females because the child is unlikely to inherit two copies of the recessive allele. This may be because the condition is rare, or because affected males are reproductively disadvantaged.

PGD for gender selection may also be used for non-Mendelian disorders that are significantly more prevalent in one sex. For the prevention of these inherited disorders, the gender of offspring is selected based on the seriousness of inherited condition, the risk ratio in either sex, and the options for disease treatment (Amor & Cameron, 2008).

"Non-medical" applications of PGD for family balancing (also known as "social sexing" or "social sex selection") are more controversial. There is no broad cultural preference for male or female offspring in the U.S., but there is a preference of males in some countries, such as China, India and the Middle East. This non-medical use of PGD for gender selection and family balancing is prohibited in many countries such as China, because it could disrupt the sex ratio of the population.

2.3.2 Method of PGD for gender selection

We have performed PGD for gender selection by WGA of single blastomeres by MDA, followed by multiplex PCR for detecting X- and Y-linked genetic loci (E.C. Lau, M.M. Janson & K. Wang, unpublished). The Medical College of Wisconsin and Froedtert Hospital do not support non-medical use of PGD. We provide PGD for gender selection to help families with X-linked disorders give birth to unaffected children.

2.3.3 Sperm separation in combination with PGD for selecting female embryos

Sperm sorting techniques prior to IVF can be combined with post-fertilization molecular diagnosis of the resulting embryos. To prevent the birth of affected children, female embryos can be selected by PGD after forming embryos through ICSI with X-bearing sperm. For families at risk for rare X-linked recessive disorders, such as Wiskott-Aldrich syndrome (WAS) and monocarboxylate transporter 8-specific thyroid hormone cell transporter (THCT) deficiency, sperm sorting can be combined with PGD for selecting female embryos instead of developing custom PGD assays for these disorders.

PGD for gender selection can also be used to increase the odds of conceiving an HLA-matched, unaffected sibling donor. For a family with an X-linked recessive disorder that has an affected child in need of a hematopoietic progenitor cell transplant from cord blood or bone marrow, the combined use of sperm sorting and PGD for gender selection increases the chance of finding an HLA-matched and unaffected sibling donor to approximately 1 in 5. Otherwise, the chance of finding an HLA-matched female embryo by PGD is only approximately 1 in 10.

2.4 PGS/PGD for cytogenetic anomalies

Preimplantation screening for cytogenetic anomalies, in particular aneuploidies and translocations, has been performed using either FISH probes or array-comparative genomic hybridization. We shall discuss the challenges and limitations of both methods.

2.4.1 Aneuploidy for whole chromosomes

The adoption of FISH in a preimplantation context was a natural adaptation of FISH techniques as used in prenatal diagnosis (PND), where its value in assessing aneuploidy is unassailable. In contrast to prenatal specimens, only single, or at most two cells, are available for preimplantation genetic testing (PGT), and thus single FISH probe cocktails must employ at least 5 fluorochromes to cover the most prevalent liveborn aneuploidies, namely, 13, 18, 21, the X and Y. The availability of commercially produced cocktails has alleviated the need to "home brew" probes, but has necessitated the acquisition of more comprehensive fluorescent filter sets than those used for most routine two- or three-color FISH.

Following biopsy of an embryo the single blastomeres are placed in a hypotonic solution, and then treated with acetic acid methanol to fix and spread the cells. All these are performed by an embryologist. Ideally this will result in a uniformly flat nucleus with little or no overlying cytoplasm. Larger swelled nuclei which have not ruptured and have therefore preserved the nuclear contents are desired in order to separate the hybridization signals, especially for the large centromere targets, 18, X and Y. Subsequent steps are performed in the cytogenetics laboratory. From this point forward a major departure from PND, where typically 50 nuclei are assessed, is the reliance on a single nucleus for aneuploidy diagnosis. Thus, there is a need for consistency in the fixation and spreading, and freedom from artifacts such as spurious extra signals or weak signals, which are inconsequential in multi-cell analyses.

The partial coverage of a 5-probe set can be partly overcome by sequential hybridizations to the same nucleus. The quality and consistency of a second or subsequent hybridization are , however, generally progressively inferior due to the damaging hot treatments at 73 °C, which are necessary for denaturation and stringent washing. Preliminary indications of commercial development of a 6-step reduced-temperature sequential hybridization strategy to cover all 24 chromosomes have not to our knowledge been realized, and routine widespread use of such a strategy may not be technically realistic.

Nevertheless, a second hybridization cycle can detect the more common aneuploidies seen in early spontaneous pregnancy losses, namely, trisomies 15, 16 and 22. An example of a home-brew second cycle is shown in Fig. 2, and utilizes a contrasting color mixture of alpha satellite for 15, alpha satellite for 16 and the BCR locus for 22.

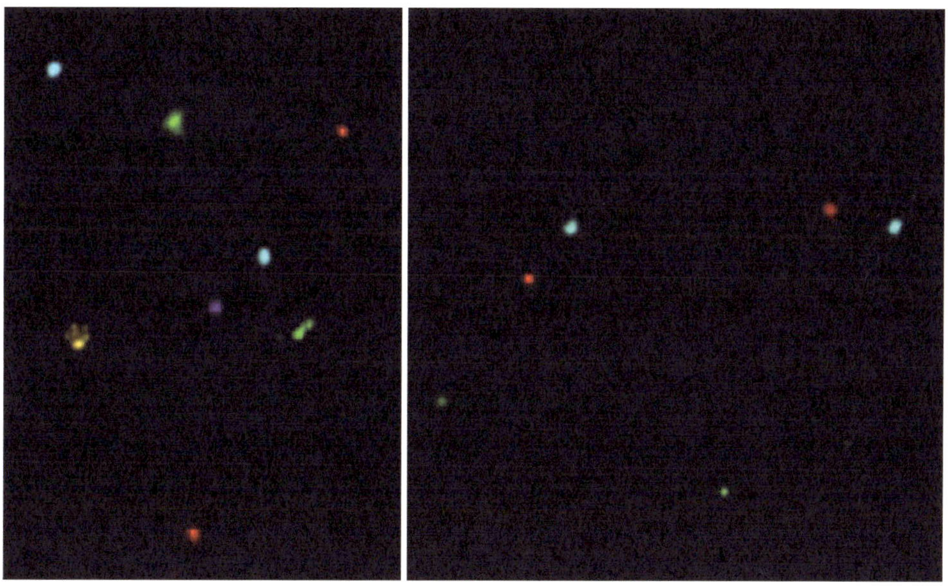

Fig. 2. Panel on left is a first cycle of hybridization using Abbott PGT cocktail. Fluorochrome scheme: red = 13, aqua = 18, green = 21, blue = X and Y = gold. This nucleus is euploid for these chromosomes and is male. Panel on right is cycle 2 of the same nucleus. Fluorochrome scheme: orange = 15, aqua = 16, green = 22, all obtained from Abbott Laboratories. The single copy unique sequence BCR is thus the smallest signal.

From the foregoing discussion one can deduce that several technical difficulties limit the usefulness of FISH in aneuploidy assessment. Due to artifactual variation in quality the clarity of results seen in Fig. 2 is not always achieved, resulting in ambiguous diagnosis or no diagnosis for an embryo. This limitation is inherent to the fact that a single data point (FISH signal) in a single nucleus is to be regarded potentially as representative of the entire embryo. Secondly, an obvious limitation is the extent of genome coverage, which often encompasses only the potentially liveborn trisomies, with a complete absence of information regarding other unsampled genomic regions.

Both these limitations are overcome by the use of genomic copy number microarrays (see Section 3 below). Firstly, each chromosome is represented by many data points by array hybridization, making 1, 2 or 3-copy number calls more statistically reliable. Secondly, all the chromosomes are represented on arrays, thus all aneupoloides leading to early pregnancy loss can be detected.

2.4.2 Aneuploidy for sub-chromosomal regions

Arrays using single-cell amplified DNA may not yet be necessarily sensitive enough to detect sub-chromosomal aneuploidy. Examples may include small extra marker chromosomes or unbalanced segregants of reciprocal translocation, both of which can lead to unfavorable pregnancy outcomes. FISH may continue to be of utility in assessing aneuploidy from translocation of small but genetically significant regions that have been associated with developmental delay or pregnancy loss. We have used a FISH strategy when the microarray service cannot provide assurance of reliable coverage of small regions.

An example in our experience is a couple which suffered two pregnancy losses due, in each case, to different unbalanced adjacent-1 meiotic segregation products. The small regions involved are shown in Fig. 3.

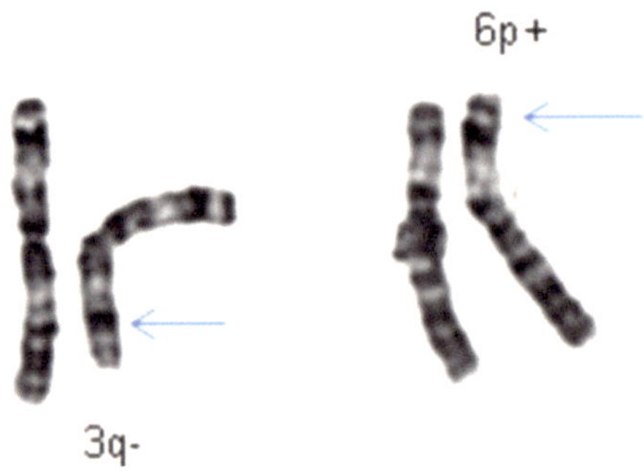

Fig. 3. Balanced t(3;6)(q25.3;p22.2) in a woman with repeated miscarriages and unbalanced pregnancy losses. Both unbalanced adjacent-1 products have been observed in karyotyped products of conception.

The probe scheme used to assess their embryos is illustrated in Fig. 4. It also illustrates the general rule that labeling three of the four arms of the quadrivalent with probes is necessary and sufficient to detect any of the 12 unbalanced products possible, including both adjacent-1, both adjacent-2 as well as all eight 3:1 segregants. An advantage of translocation FISH over aneuploid FISH is that often two data points will mark an unbalanced meiotic product, since all adjacent-2 and half of 3:1 products result in a duplication or deficiency for two probes. This strategy has been adopted in three pregnancy cycles in the aforementioned couple.

FISH patterns from an embryo clearly unbalanced with an extra 3p signal but a single 6 centromere are shown in Fig. 5a. This is interpreted as an adjacent-2 segregant, cartooned in Fig. 5b. This would result in 3 copies for most of 3 and monosomy for most of 6.

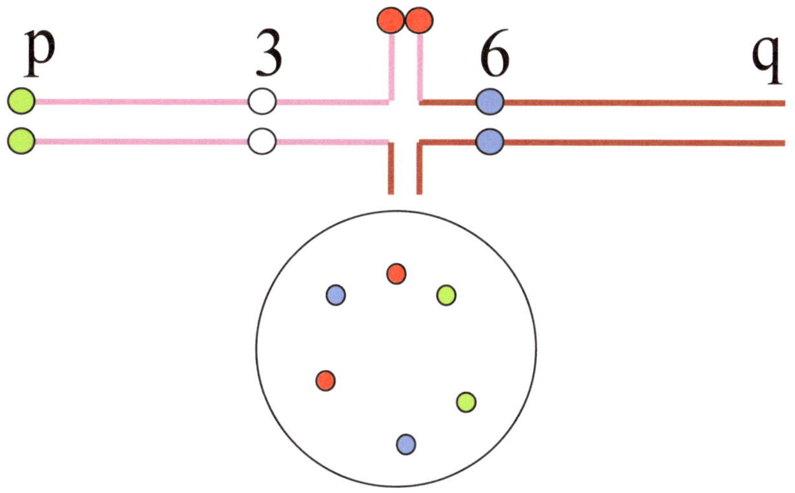

Fig. 4. *Top,* scheme to detect unbalanced t(3;6) meiotic products: subtelomere green (3p) and orange (3q) as well as 6 centromere (aqua). Three contrasting probes are sufficient to detect all unbalanced products. *Bottom,* this interphase pattern is balanced, any other pattern is unbalanced, following fertilization.

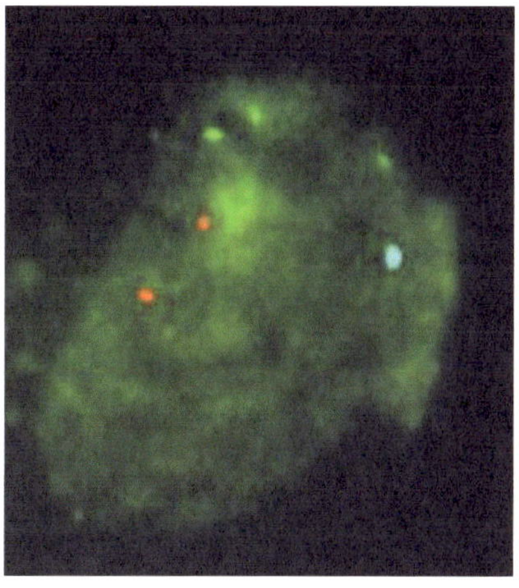

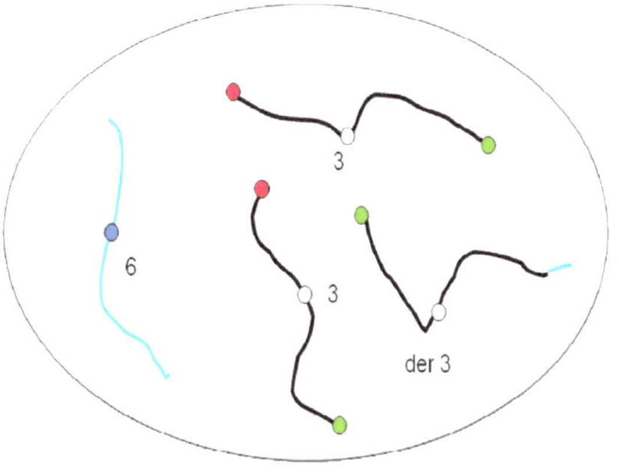

Fig. 5. *Left,* shows FISH patterns with an extra 3p signal and deficient for a 6 centromere signal. This is one of two cells from this embryo showing adjacent-2 segregation. *Right,* depicts this unbalanced complement.

To date adjacent-1 and adjacent-2 segregants have been detected in this couple, including those equivalent to both of the previous cytogenetically documented pregnancy losses.

It should be emphasized that both FISH and microarray approaches are limited in predictive value by strictly biological considerations. It is apparent by numerous studies that many early embryos are mosaic for aneuploidy. In addition, mosaic embryos often "correct", leading to normal outcomes following an aneuploid finding based on a single cell (Barbash-Hazan et al, 2009). Thus, both false negative and false positive findings may be expected from these single cell approaches. These considerations must be kept in mind when counseling couples to the value and accuracy of anueploid PGD.

3. Technological advances in preimplantation genetic testing

Robust WGA protocols (see section 2.2 above) and high-throughput DNA technologies such as microarrays and next generation sequencing (NGS) make it reasonable to envision PGD by interrogating the complete genome of a single blastomere. Completing a whole-genome analysis within the time frame of an IVF cycle via either technology remains a technical challenge. Genomic strategies, however, offer the promise of universal diagnosis and screening methods with consequent advantages in cost efficiency and diagnostic power. Emerging technologies for whole genome analysis via DNA microarrays and DNA sequencing are rapidly becoming more powerful and more cost effective, and it will soon be feasible to apply these genomic tools widely in reproductive medicine.

3.1 PGD/PGS by microarrays

DNA microarray technologies measure hybridization between the subject's DNA (the "target") and a matrix of known DNA sequences (the array "features") immobilized on a solid state matrix. Depending upon the array platform and hybridization protocol, microarrays can reveal gains or losses of genome segments or determine the subject's genotype for SNPs.

Array-comparative genomic hybridization (aCGH) has become an established alternative to FISH for PGS of aneuploidies, unbalanced translocations and complex karyotypes with multiple rearrangements (Hellani et al., 2008; Van den Veyver et al., 2009; Harper & Harton, 2010; Alfarawati et al., 2011; Fiorentino et al., 2011; Vanneste et al., 2011). In this procedure, target and control genomic DNAs are mixed and competitively hybridized to the same array. Changes in the hybridization ratio of target to control at a region indicate a gain or loss of material relative to the control genome. Since aCGH interrogates every chromosome and reveals events below the limits of microscopic detection, it is able to identify chromosome anomalies that a standard 8- or 12-chromosome FISH might fail to detect. However, aCGH does not detect balanced rearrangements or triploidy, where the target:control DNAs hybridized to the array features is constant along the genome (Thornhill et al., 2008; Harper & Harton, 2010; Fiorentino et al., 2011).

Single-gene disorders are amenable to whole-genome analysis using SNP microarrays. The SNP array features include alternative alleles for a large number of polymorphisms, and hybridization indicates which SNP allele(s) are present in the target genome. The SNP genotypes of two parents and a reference child define maternal and paternal haplotypes at a gene of interest, and linkage then establishes the genetic risk for a second child based on its combination of parental haplotypes. The analysis is similar to STR haplotyping discussed previously (see section 2.2.2). While custom PGD linkage assays have been developed for less than 10% of the known single gene disorders, a single microarray generates predictive SNP haplotypes for the entire genome.

Handyside et al. (2010) employed SNP genotype data to create "karyomaps" that represent the parental haplotypes and points of recombination along a child's chromosomes. In this work, SNP haplotypes were shown to coincide with the inheritance of cystic fibrosis in families where both parents were carriers for CFTR mutations (Handyside et al., 2010).

Unpublished results from our laboratory (C.B. Ball & E.C. Lau) also serve as support the concept of SNP haplotyping for Mendelian disorders. SNP haplotypes linked to eleven loci of clinical interest were analyzed in a family of four individuals. At each locus, a region comprised of the gene of interest and 2 Mb flanking on either side contained sufficient informative SNPs to infer paternal and maternal haplotypes and predict the genetic status of a sibling to the reference child. We validated the SNP haplotypes analysis with PCR assays for STRs linked to three of the eleven loci (see section 2.2.2). Table 1 (a and b) summarizes the findings for these three genes:

(a) SNP haplotypes linked to loci of interest and diagnosis for proband child.

Locus	Linked SNPs		SNP Haplotypes				# of SNPs matching proband call
	Total	Informative	Father	Mother	Reference child	Proband child	
CFTR	903	255	P1 P2	M1 M2	P1 M1	P2 M2	245 / 253
HBB	1,747	528	P1 P2	M1 M2	P1 M1	P1 M2	499 / 528
PKHD1	1,492	488	P1 P2	M1 M2	P1 M1	P1 M2	472 / 488

(b) STR haplotypes linked to loci of interest and diagnosis for proband child.

Locus	STR location	STR haplotypes STR allele sizes in bp			
		Father	Mother	Reference child	Proband child
CFTR	3′ flanking region	P1 P2 211, 204	M1 M2 204, 231	P1 M1 211, 204	P2 M2 204, 231
HBB	5′ flanking region	P1 P2 137, 141	M1 M2 127, 119	P1 M1 137, 127	P1 M2 137. 119
PKHD1	5′ flanking region	P1 P2 348, 363	M1 M2 352, 344	P1 M1 348, 352	P1 M2 348, 344
	intragenic	P1 P2 254, 260	M1 M2 260, 264	P1 M1 254, 260	P1 M2 254, 264
	3′ flanking region	P1 P2 232, 228	M1 M2 230, 228	P1 M1 232, 230	P1 M2 232, 228

Table 1. Comparison of haplotyping for SNPs linked to three clinically significant loci (a) with haplotyping for STRs linked to the same loci (b).

It should be noted that of 21 custom primers tested, only five assays were informative in this pedigree (Table 1b). This illustrates the universality of SNP genotyping compared to STR methods and the value of avoiding custom assays.

SNP arrays are also of value in assessing aneuploidy and unbalanced chromosome rearrangements. Johnson et al. (2010) showed that integrating SNP genotype data with copy number improved the quality of analysis for noisy data such as those obtained from single-cell WGA. Similarly, Handyside et al. (2011) established that karyomapping across the whole genome would detect chromosome imbalances and identify the parent of origin for the imbalance based on the parental genotypes.

3.2 Future PGD/PGS by DNA sequencing

Besides high-density microarrays, SNPs can be detected genome-wide by DNA sequencing, which provides genotyping analysis at the highest resolution. For PGD of single-gene disorders, DNA sequencing would be the future method of choice. The assay can interrogate the entire genome, or target specific regions and genes of special interest. In principle, sequencing methods can search directly for a targeted base change, or generate SNP haplotypes for a linkage-based diagnosis. Second-generation sequencing systems, such as Roche 454 system, Illumina sequencers and ABI SOLiD system, have not been used for PGD due to the high cost and slow turn-around-time.

Even if the cost of whole genome DNA sequencing falls to $1,000, it is still too costly for routine clinical PGD when the total cost of sequencing the parental samples, affected child and several embryos is considered. In contrast to accurately determining the genotypes of every SNP that requires sequencing at high genome coverage, it may lower the cost of PGD using a haplotying approach that would require a lower genome coverage to identify the SNP haplotypes of embryos for transfer.

The recently released third-generation DNA sequencers, such as the Single-Molecular Real-Time System RS (Pacific Biosciences, CA), has enabled more rapid and cost effective genomic sequencing. Future sequencing technologies, such as DNA transistor nanopore sequencing system (Roche-IBM), and DNA tunneling silicon nanopore sequencer, will benefit PGD when the sequencing cost falls below $250, and the turn-around-time to be less than 24 hours.

4. Genetic counseling for PGD/PGS

Genetic counseling is an essential step for patients contemplating PGD (Swanson et al., 2007). During the counseling session information is gathered including the patient's medical and reproductive history, the partner's medical and reproductive history, and their family histories. Both the patient and her partner should attend the counseling session. If an indication of risk is not covered, it is essential that the counselor obtains the physician and/or laboratory records supporting the information. Preimplantation genetic testing should not be undertaken without a firm diagnosis. With this information in hand the counselor can discuss disorder(s) in the family, the severity and variability of such condition(s), limitations of genotype/phenotype and the patient's probability of affected children. All of this information will help a patient decide whether PGD would be a reasonable option for her situation.

If PGD appears to be an option, then information is provided detailing the testing that can be carried out on single embryonic cells. Limitations of such testing are discussed including the patient's anticipated success rate for IVF with PGD and the possibility of both false positive and false negative PGD results. Prenatal testing through chorionic villus sampling (CVS) or amniocentesis is recommended to confirm the results of PGD. Patients should be reminded of alternative reproductive options including use of donor gametes, prenatal diagnosis (PND), accepting genetic risk without further testing, adoption, and having no children or no additional children (Harton et al., 2011c).

By combining the information from the reproductive medicine specialist and the genetic counselor, the patient can decide whether to pursue PGD. It is important that the counseling provided should be non-directive, to enable the patient to reach her own conclusion about the suitability of PGD (Shenfield et al., 2003).

5. Future prospects for preimplantation genetic diagnosis

Severe genetic disorders are debilitating, expensive and incurable conditions. The patient, the family and society at large each have an interest in avoiding the birth of a child with such a disease. PGD provides that option in a cost-effective manner, without resort to termination of an affected pregnancy.

5.1 Current status of choice between PGD/PGS and PND in the U.S.

Prenatal diagnosis (PND) of fetuses is performed by either amniocentesis or CVS performed at different stages of fetal development, but the procedures are invasive and parents may ultimately decide to terminate an affected fetus. Even though PGD has been available for 21 years, PND following natural conception still prevails in the U.S. For couples at risk of severe inherited genetic disorders, abortion of affected pregnancy is still the most common option, especially in those States which do not have mandatory insurance coverage for IVF and PGD.

5.2 Medical and economic considerations of universal access to PGD/PGS

The medical community has recently begun to address the medical and economic implications of implementing a national PGD program to help couples who are carriers of severe single-gene disorders.

About 1000 children affected with cystic fibrosis (CF) are born annually in the U.S., in some part due to reluctance to terminate affected pregnancies. There is the potential to save 33 billion dollars in lifetime medical care for those affected with this disorder if carrier parents had the option of undergoing government-backed or insurance-mandated PGD and IVF (Tur-Kaspa et al., 2010). For couples who are carriers of severe inherited genetic disorders, prevention of affected pregnancy by PGD may be a preferred option to the termination of affected fetuses (Davis et al., 2009). Thus, economic and medical considerations favor a universal and affordable access to IVF, PGD or PGS services for carrier couples of severe single-gene disorders such as CF, or for individuals at risk for transmitting chromosomal translocations, but cannot afford it (Handyside, 2010).

6. Ethical concerns

The non-medical use of PGD and PGS presents some ethical concerns. While PGD has mainly been used to select embryos unaffected with severe genetic diseases to avoid the transmission of some medical conditions, PGD may also have the potential to select an embryo affected with the same disability or disease that affects the parents, such as deafness. A deaf child born to a deaf couple would be better suited to the parents' shared culture.

There is resistance regarding the practice of reproductive technologies including IVF, PND, abortion, sperm sorting, PGD/PGS, and embryonic stem cells. In fact, many countries have banned the use of PGD for gender selection, but it is permitted in the U.S. The opponents of "social sex selection" argue that the consequences of preimplantation procedures such as sperm sorting, PGD and PGS would artificially unequalize the ratio of females to males. The opponents of PGD and PGS fear that these technologies could be used for eugenic purposes, or increasing uses of PGD may open the door to other eugenic technologies.

PGD has successfully been used to prevent the transmission of single-gene disorders with Mendelian inheritance, but has not been used for complex genetic disorders because there is insufficient amount of amplified DNA from a single blastomere with high fidelity for testing a large number of genes and single-nucleotide polymorphisms (SNPs). Complex genetic disorders (e.g. diabetes mellitus), athletic ability and intelligence are controlled by many genes and environmental factors. Similarly, physical traits (e.g. body height), and cosmetic traits (e.g. hair color, eye color and skin pigmentation) are determined by multiple genes and SNPs (Sulem et al., 2007). With the recent advancement in blastocyst biopsy for removing multiple cells, cryopreservation of blastocysts, whole-genome amplification methods that generate amplified DNA with high fidelity, it has been technically feasible to provide preimplantation testing for complex genetic disorders and human traits. When PGD expands its scope to such a non-medical realm in potential attempts to make "designer babies", it will spark more debates and controversy that might lead to legislation in this area.

7. Conclusion

Preimplantation genetic testing is an important application of IVF and has broad interest to reproductive medicine practitioners. Economic and medical considerations favor a universal and affordable access to IVF and PGD/PGS services for carrier couples of severe inherited genetic disorders. In addition to current methodologies, preimplantation testing is an expanding field poised to adopt cutting-edge genomic technologies for new advances in preventative medical care. Technologies for interrogating whole genomes via via SNP microarrays microarrays and DNA sequencing are rapidly becoming more powerful and more cost-effective. It will soon be feasible to apply these genomic tools widely in reproductive medicine.

8. Acknowledgments

The authors gratefully acknowledge the excellent support of our colleagues in the PGD team Amy Granlund, Bridget Lawler, Barbara Szlendakova and Julie McCarrier.

9. References

Alfarawati, S.; Fragouli, E.; Colls, P. & Wells, D. (2011) First births after preimplantation genetic diagnosis of structural chromosome abnormalities using comparative genomic hybridization and microarray analysis. *Human Reproduction,* Vol 26, No. 6, pp. 1560-1574.

Altarescu, G.; Geva, T.E.; Brooks, B.; Margalioth, E.; Levy-Lahad, E. & Renbaum, P. (2008). PGD on a recombinant allele: crossover between the TSC2 gene and 'linked' markers impairs accurate diagnosis. *Prenatal Diagnosis,* Vol.28, No.10, pp. 929-933.

Amor, D.J. & Cameron, C. PGD gender selection for non-Mendelian disorders with unequal sex incidence. (2008). *Human Reproduction,* Vol.23, No.4, pp. 729-734.

Amos, J.; Feldman, G.L.; Grody, W.W.; Monaghan, K.; Palomaki, G.E.; Prior, T.W.; Richards, C.S & Watson, M.S. (2006). Technical standards and guidelines for CFTR mutation testing 2006 edition. Available from http://www.acmg.net/Pages/ACMG_Activities/stds-2002/cf.htm

Barbash-Hazan, S.; Frumkin, T.; Malcov, M.; Yaron, Y.; Cohen, T.; Azern, F.; Amit, A. & Ben-Yosef, D. (2009). Preimplantation aneuploid embryos undergo self-correction in correlation with their developmental potential. *Fertility & Sterility,* Vol.92, No.3, pp. 890-896.

Bick, D.P. & Lau, E.C. (2006). Preimplantation genetic diagnosis. *Pediatric Clinics of North America,* Vol.53, No.4, pp. 559-577.

Bick, S.L.; Bick, B.P.; Wells, B.E.; Roesler, M.R.; Strawn, E.Y. & Lau, E.C. (2008). Preimplantation HLA haplotyping using tri-, tetra-, and pentanucleotide short tandem repeats for HLA matching. *Journal of Assisted Reproduction and Genetics,* Vol.25, pp. 323-331.

Benson, J.B. & Haith, M.M. (2009). *Diseases and Disorders in Infancy and Early Childhood.* Academic Press,. p. 210.

Coskun, S. & Alsmadi, O. (2007). Whole genome amplification from a single cell: a new era for preimplantation genetic diagnosis. *Prenatal Diagnosis,* Vol.27, pp. 297-302.

Cooper, A.R. & Jungheim E.S. (2010). Preimplantation genetic testing: indications and controversies. *Clinical Laboratory Medicine,* Vol.30, No.3, pp. 519-531.

Daniels G.; Pettigrew R.; Thornhill A.; Abbs S.; Lashwood A.; O'Mahony F. et al. (2001). Six unaffected livebirths following preimplantation diagnostic for spinal muscular atrophy. *Moleclar Human Reproduction,* Vol.7, No.10, pp. 995-1000.

Davis, L.B.; Champion, S.J.; Fair, S.Q.; Baker, V.L. & Garber, A.M. (2009). A cost-benefit analysis of preimplantation genetic diagnosis for carrier couples of cystic fibrosis. *Fertility & Sterility,* Vol.93, No.6, pp. 1793-1804.

Dean, F.B.; Hosono, S.; Fang, L.; Wu, X.; Faruqi, A.F.; Bray-Ward, P. et al. (2002). Comprehensive human genome amplification using multiple displacement amplification. *Proceedings of the National Academy of Sciences USA,* Vol.99, pp. 5261-5266.

Dell, K.M. & Avner, E.D. (July 2008). Autosomal recessive polycystic kidney disease. In: *Gene Reviews,* NIH, NCBI Bookshelf Available from: http://www.ncbi.nlm.nih.gov/books/NBK1326/.

ESHRE PGD Consortium Steering Committee. (2002). ESHRE Preimplantation Genetic Diagnosis Consortium: data collection III (May 2001). *Human Reproduction,* Vol.17, No.1, pp.233-246.

Fiorentino, F.; Spizzichino, L.; Bono, S.; Biricik, A.; Kokkali, G.; Rienzi, L. et al. (2011). PGD for reciprocal and Robertsonian translocations using array comparative genomic hybridization. *Human Reproduction,* Vol.26, No.7, pp. 1925-1935.

Grewal, S.S.; Kahn, J.P.; MacMillan, M.L;, Ramsay, N.K & Wagner, J.E. (2004). Successful hematopoietic stem cell transplantation for Fanconi anemia from an unaffected HLA-genotype-identical sibling selected using preimplantation genetic diagnosis. *Blood,* Vol.103, pp. 1147-1151.

Handyside, A.H. (2010). Preimplantation genetic diagnosis after 20 years. *Reproductive BioMedicine Online,* Vol.21, No.3, pp. 280-282.

Handyside, A.H.; Kontogianni, E.H.; Hardy, K. & Winston, R.M. (1990). Pregnancies from biopsied human preimplantation embryos sexed by Y-specific DNA amplification. *Nature,* Vol.344, pp. 768-770.

Handyside, A.H.; Lesko, J.G.; Tarin, J.J.; Winston, R.M. & Hughes, M.R. (1992). Birth of a normal girl after in vitro fertilization and preimplantation diagnostic testing for cystic fibrosis. *The New England Journal of Medicine, Vol.*327, pp. 905-909.

Handyside, A.H.; Harton, G.L.; Mariani, B.; Thornhill, A.R.; Affara, N.; Shaw, M-A & Griffin, D.K. (2010). Karyomapping: a universal method for genome wide analysis of genetic disease based on mapping crossovers between parental haplotypes. *Journal of Medical Genetics,* Vol.47, No.10, pp. 651-658.

Handyside, A.H.; Robinson, M.D.; Simpson, R.J.; Omar, M.B.; Shaw, M.-A.; Grudzinskas, J.G. et al. (2004). Isothermal whole genome amplification from single and small numbers of cells: a new era for preimplantation genetic diagnosis of inherited disease. *Molecular Human Reproduction,* Vol.10, No.10, pp. 767-772.

Harper, J.C. & Harton, G.L. (2010) The use of arrays in preimplantation genetic diagnosis and screening. *Fertility and Sterility,* Vol.10, No.4, pp.1173-1177.

Harper, J.C.; Coonen, E.; De Rycke, M.; Harton, G.; Moutou, C.; Pehlivans, T.; Traeger-Synodinos, J.; Van Rij, M.C. & Goossens, V. (2010). ESHRE PGS Consortium data collection X: cycles from January to December 2007 with pregnancy followup to October 2008. *Human Reproduction,* Vol.25, No.11, pp.2685-2707.

Harton, G.L.; De Rycke, M.; Fiorentino, .F.; Moutou, C.; SenGupta, S.; Traeger-Synodinos, J. & Harper J.C. (2011a). ESHRE PGD consortium best practice guidelines for amplification-based PGD. *Human Reproduction,* Vol.26, pp. 33-40.

Harton, G.L.; Magli, M.C.; Lundin, K.; Montag, M.; Lemmen, J. & Harper J.C. (2011b). ESHRE PGD Consortium/Embryology Special Interest Group - best practice guidelines for polar body and embryo biopsy for preimplantation genetic diagnosis/screening (PGD/PGS). *Human Reproduction,* Vol.26, pp. 41-46.

Harton, G.; Braude, P.; Lashwood, A.; Schmutzler, A.; Traeger-Synodinos, J.; Wilton, L. & Harper, J.C. (2011c). ESHRE PGD consortium best practice guidelines for organization of a PGD centre for PGD/preimplantation genetic screening. *Human Reproduction,* Vol.26, pp. 14-24.

Heinrich, M.; Braun, T.; Sanger, T.; Saukko, P.; Lutz-Bonengel, S. & Schmidt, U. (2009). Reduced-volume and low-volume typing of Y-chromosomal SNPs to obtain Finnish Y-chromosomal compound haplotypes. *International Journal of Legal Medicine,* Vol.123, pp. 413-418.

Hellani, A.; Abu-Amero, K.; Azouri, J. & El-Akoum, S. (2008). Successful pregnancies after application of array-comparative genomic hybridization in PGS-aneuploidy screening. *Reproductive BioMedicine Online,* Vol.17, pp. 841-847.

Hellani, A.; Coskun, S.; Benkhalifa, M.; Tbakhi, A.; Sakati, N.; Al-Odaib, A. & Ozand, P. (2004). Multiple displacement amplification on single cell and possible PGD applications. *Molecular Human Reproduction,* Vol.10, pp. 847-852.

Johnson, D.S.; Gemelos, G.; Baner, J.; Ryan, A.; Cinnioglu, C.; Banjevic, M.; Ross, R. et al. (2010). Preclinical validation of a microarray method for full molecular karyotyping of blastomeres in a 24-h protocol. *Human Reproduction,* Vol.25, pp. 1066-1075.

Kobayashi, M.; Rappaport, E.; Blasband, A.; Semeraro, A.; Sartore, M.; Surrey, S. & Fortina, P. (1995). Fluorescence-based DNA minisequence analysis for detection of known single-base changes in genomic DNA. *Molecular and Cellular Probes,* Vol.9, pp. 175-182.

Lau, E.C.; Janson, M.M.; Roesler, M.R.; Avner, E.D.; Strawn, E.Y. & Bick, D.P. (2010). Birth of a healthy infant following preimplantation PKHD1 haplotyping for autosomal recessive kidney disease using multiple displacement amplification. *Journal of Assisted Reproduction and Genetics,* Vol.27, pp. 397-407.

Langmore, J.P. (2002). Rubicon Genomics, Inc. *Pharmacogenomics,* Vol.3, pp. 557-560.

Magli, M.C.; Gianaroli ,L.; Grievo, N.; Cefalu, E.; Ruvolo, G. & Ferraretti, A.P. (2006). Cryopreservation of biopsied embryos at the blastocyst stage. *Human Reproduction,* Vol.21, No.10, pp. 2656-2660.

Malcov M.; Schwartz T.; Mei-Raz N.; Yosef D.B.; Amit A.; Lessing J.B. et al. (2004). Multiplex nested PCR for preimplantation genetic diagnosis of spinal muscular atrophy. *Fetal Diagnosis and Therapy,* Vol.19, No.2, pp. 199-206.

Munne, S.; Weier, H.U.; Stein, J.; Grifo, J. & Cohen, J. (1993). A fast and efficient method for simultaneous X and Y in situ hybridization of human blastomeres. *Journal of Assisted Reproduction and Genetics,* Vol.10, pp. 82-90.

Munne, S.; Scott, R.; Sable, D. & Cohen, J. (1998). First pregnancies after preconception diagnosis of translocations of maternal origin. *Fertility and Sterility,* Vol.69, pp. 675-681.

Palermo, G.; Joris, H.; Devroey, P. & Van Steirteghem, A.C. (1992). Pregnancies after intracytoplasmic injection of single spermatozoon into an oozyte. *Lancet,* Vol.340, pp. 17-18.

Prior, T.W. & Russman, B.S. (2011). Spinal Muscular Atrophy, In: *GeneReviews,* Available from http://www.ncbi.nlm.nih.gov/books/NBK1352/

Schrurs, B.M.; Winston, R.M. & Handyside, A.H. (1993). Preimplantation diagnosis of aneuploidy using fluorescent in-situ hybridization: evaluation using a chromosome 18-specific probe. *Human Reproduction,* Vol.8, pp. 296-301.

Sermon, K.; Lissens, W.; Joris, H.; Van Steirteghem, A. & Liebaers, I. (1996). Adaptation of the primer extension preimplantation (PEP) reaction for preimplantation diagnosis: single blastomere analysis using short PEP protocols. *Molecular Human Reproduction,* Vol.2, pp. 209-212.

Shenfield, F.; Pennings, G.; Devroey, P.; Sureau, C.; Tarlatzis, B. & Cohen, J. (2003). Taskforce 5: preimplantation genetic diagnosis. *Human Reproduction,* Vol.18, No.3, pp. 649-651.

Stachecki, J.J.; Cohen, J. & Munne, S. (2005). Cryopreservation of biopsied cleavage stage human embryos. *Reproductive BioMedicine Online,* Vol.11, No.6, pp. 711-715.

Sulem, P.; Gudbjartsson, D.F.; Stacey, S.N.; Helgason A.; Rafnar, T.; Magnusson, K.P. et al. (2007). Genetic determinants of hair, eye and skin pigmentation in Europeans. *Nature Genetics,* Vol.39, pp.1443-1452.

Swanson, A.; Strawn, E.; Lau, E. & Bick, D. (2007). Preimplantation genetic diagnosis: technology and clinical applications. *Wisconsin Medical Journal,* Vol.106, No.3, pp. 145-151.

Sweeney, W.E. & Avner E.D. (2006). Molecular and cellular pathophysiology of autosomal recessive polycystic kidney disease. *Cell and Tissue Research,* Vol.326, pp. 671-685.

Theisen, A. & Shaffer, L.G. (2010). Disorders caused by chromosome abnormalities. The Application of Clinical Genetics, Vol.2010, No.3, pp.159-174.

Thornhill, A.R.; Gabriel, A.S.; Gordon, A.; Griffin, D.K.; Taylor, J. & Handyside, A.H. (2008). Array CGH for use in clinical preimplantation genetic screening. *Fertility and Sterility*, Vol.90 supplement, p. S306.

Tur-Kaspa, I.; Aljadeff, G.; Rechitsky, S.; Grotjan, H.E. & Verlinsky, Y. (2010). PGD for all cystic fibrosis carrier couples: novel strategy for preventive medicine and cost analysis. *Reproductive BioMedicine Online, Vol.*21, No.2, pp. 186-195.

Vanneste, E.; Melotte, C.; Voetl, T; Robberecth, C.; Debrock, S.; Pexsters, A.; Staessen, C.; Tomassetti, C.; Legius, E.; D'Hooghe, T. & Vermeesch, J.R. (2011). PGD for a complex chromosomal rearrangement by array comparative genomic hybridization. *Human Reproduction*, Vol.26, No.4, pp.941-949.

Van den Veyver, I.B.; Patel, A.; Shaw, C.; Pursley, A.N.; Kang, S. L.; Simovitch, M.J.; Ward, P.A.; Darilek, S.; Johnson, A.; Neill, S.E.; Bi, W.; White, L.D., Eng, C.M. , Lupski, J.R.; Cheung, S.W. & Beaudet, A.L. (2009). Clinical use of array comparative genomic hybridization (aCGH) for prenatal diagnosis in 300 cases. *Prenatal Diagnosis*, Vol.29, No.1, pp.29-39.

Verlinsky, Y.; Cohen, J.; Munne, S.; Gianaroli, L.; Simpson, J.L.; Ferraretti, A.P. & Kuliev, A. (2004). Over a decade of experience with preimplantation genetic diagnosis: a multicenter report. *Fertility & Sterility,* Vol.82, No.2, pp.292-294.

Verlinsky, Y.; Rechitsky, S.; Schoolcraft, W.; Strom, C. & Kuliev, A. (2001). Preimplantation diagnosis for Fanconi anemia combined with HLA matching. *The Journal of the American Medical Association,* Vol.285, pp. 3130-3133.

Zhang, L.; Cui, X.; Schmitt, K.; Hubert, R.; Navidi, W. & Arnheim, N. (1992). Whole genome amplification from a single cell: implications for genetic analysis. *The Proceedings of National Academy of Sciences,* Vol.89, pp. 5847-5851.

Zhang, X.; Trokoudes, K.M. & Pavlides, C. (2009).Vitrification of biopsied embryos at cleavage, morula and blastocyst stage.. *Reproductive BioMedicine Online,* Vol.19, No.4, pp. 526-531.

Zheng, W.T.; Zhuang, G.L.; Zhou, C.Q.; Fang, C.; Ou, J.P.; Li, T.; Zhang, M.F. & Liang, X.Y. (2005). Comparison of the survival of human biopsied embryos after cryopreservation with four different methods using non-transferable embryos. *Human Reproduction,* Vol.20, No.6, pp. 1615-1618.